Current Issues
in
Clinical Lactation

2002

Kathleen G. Auerbach

Current Issues
in
Clinical Lactation

2002

Kathleen G. Auerbach

JONES AND BARTLETT PUBLISHERS

Sudbury, Massachusetts

BOSTON   TORONTO   LONDON   SINGAPORE

World Headquarters

Jones and Bartlett Publishers
40 Tall Pine Drive
Sudbury, MA 01776
978-443-5000
info@jbpub.com
www.jbpub.com

Jones and Bartlett Publishers Canada
2100 Bloor Street West
Suite 6-272
Toronto, ON M6S 5A5
CANADA

Jones and Bartlett Publishers International
Barb House, Barb Mews
London W6 7PA
UK

Production Credits:
Acquisitions Editor: Penny Glynn
Production Editor: Elizabeth Platt
Director of Manufacturing: Therese Bräuer
Cover Design: Anne Spencer
Printing and Binding: Malloy Lithographing

CIP data unavailable at time of printing

0-7637-1822-x

Printed in the United States of America

Current Issues in
Clinical Lactation
2002

Table of Contents

Current Issues In Clinical Lactation 2002

Editor
Kathleen G. Auerbach, PhD, IBCLC
Ferndale, Washington USA

Associate Editor
Mary-Margaret Coates, MS, IBCLC
Wheat Ridge, Colorado USA

Contributing Editors
Pat Martens, PhD, IBCLC
Winnipeg, Manitoba, Canada

Diane Wiessinger, MS, IBCLC
Ithaca, New York USA

Barbara Wilson-Clay, BSEd, IBCLC
Manchaca, Texas USA

From the Editor

Of Differences and Similarities

Kathleen G. Auerbach, PhD, IBCLC

Kathleen G. Auerbach is Editor-in-Chief of *CICL*. She maintains a private practice in lactation consulting at The Parent Center (Ferndale, WA USA), and is co-author with Jan Riordan of *Breastfeeding and Human Lactation* and four accompanying titles. Contact the author at 6145 N. Beulah Avenue, Ferndale, WA 98248 USA.

Current Issues in Clinical Lactation, 2002, 1–2; differences, similarities.

Every publication has its own flavor. Sometimes its subject matter is clearly informed through the title. In other cases, the reader may find a more subtle topic through a clustering of articles of similar topics. In this publication, you will find a variety of topics and—if you look carefully—some similarities.

We have included a commentary (Mennella, pp. 3–9) discussing research findings that represents both old and new information. Furthermore, it provides cautions for the lactation professional to consider when working with women for whom questions about alcohol consumption may not have been fully addressed. Buckley (pp. 23–35) describes differences in views about extended breastfeeding in two ethnic groups, suggesting that how health providers view breastfeeding may confer negative messages to women considering breastfeeding beyond one year postpartum.

In two different columns, you will find information relating to the care and assistance of preterm infants and their mothers (Piper, pp. 11–21; Mercer, pp. 49–53). See also Hewat's commentary and plea for extended support for these mother-baby pairs (pp. 55–57). Even if you see only full-term, healthy neonates, these articles may offer important insights you can use.

Wilson-Clay and Maloney (pp. 59–67) offer a means of fostering and maintaining communication between hospital-based and community-based clinicians who see and assist the same client. And, Wiessinger (pp. 69–73) highlights the importance of Step 10 for the breastfeeding mother who goes home from the hospital to a non-supportive culture. Her suggestion that this may be the most important of the Ten Steps dovetails with Wilson-Clay and Maloney's column without these authors having discussed the focus of their respective discussions in advance!

In still another column, Martens (pp. 37–47) discusses the many ways in which research findings can be contaminated by bias. The most important bias of all—one almost never discussed formally—relates to those biases we, as readers and clinicians, bring to the table when reading research papers and seeking to incorporate their findings in our daily work. Her discussion points out the importance of reading critically and acting cautiously when applying those findings to our clinical practices.

In short, this publication is a *potpourri* of quite different, yet simultaneously similar, discussions. We hope that their differences as well as their similarities provoke thought and serious informed discussion with your peers. In fact, we challenge you to tell us how you *use* these articles.

Commentary

Alcohol Use During Lactation:
The Folklore Versus the Science

Julie A. Mennella, PhD

Julie Mennella is a Member of the Monell Chemical Senses Center, Philadelphia, Pennsylvania USA. This research was supported by Grant AA09523 from the National Institute on Alcohol Abuse and Alcoholism and the Office of Research on Women's Health. Contact the author at Monell Chemical Senses Center, 3500 Market Street, Philadelphia, PA 19104-3308 USA.

Current Issues in Clinical Lactation 2002, 3–9; alcohol, breastmilk, folklore, infant, lactation, nutrition.

Abstract

For centuries, alcohol has been recommended to breastfeeding mothers as an aid to lactation. Folklore related that drinking a small quantity of alcohol shortly before breastfeeding increased milk yield, facilitated milk letdown, and relaxed both the mother and infant. Our study found that these beliefs continue to be ingrained in current-day medical practice. We surveyed 410 lactating women living in the

For centuries, alcohol has been recommended to lactating women as an aid to lactation.

Delaware Valley about the type of advice, if any, that they received about alcohol use during pregnancy and lactation. Twenty-five percent of the women reported that a health professional encouraged them to drink alcohol; approximately half of the women (54%) reported receiving no advice at all; and the remainder (nearly 21%) was advised to refrain from drinking. Of particular interest is the finding that 23% of the women whose health professionals discouraged them from drinking alcohol while they were pregnant were encouraged to drink when they began lactating. In this article, I review the research, albeit limited, on the transfer of alcohol to human milk and its effect on the nursing mother and her suckling infant. Based on this science, the recommendation for a breastfeeding mother to drink a glass of beer or wine shortly before nursing may be counterproductive. While mothers may be more relaxed after a drink, their babies will ingest less milk and their sleep may be disrupted.

Introduction

Traditionally, alcohol has been recommended to breast-feeding mothers as an aid to lactation. Some physicians in the early 19th century counseled abstinence because they believed that the most frequent source of acquired alcoholism was exposure to alcohol in mothers' milk (Robinovitch, 1903; Routh, 1879). Folklore related that drinking small quantities of alcohol shortly before nursing increased milk yield, facilitated milk letdown, and relaxed both mother and infant. These beliefs about alcohol's benefits for

lactating women are remarkably reminiscent of those for pregnant women (see Davidson, et al, 1981) prior to the scientific and clinical investigations on the effects of prenatal alcohol exposure. That is, "there are no dangers and it is good for you and your baby!" This folklore was so well ingrained in American tradition that, in 1895, a major US brewery produced a low alcoholic beer composed of barley malt and hops. It was sold exclusively in drugstores and prescribed by physicians as a tonic for pregnant and breastfeeding women and as a nutritional beverage for children (Krebs, 1953). Its production was halted during Prohibition because it contained more than 0.5% alcohol.

Nearly a quarter of the lactating women surveyed reported that they were encouraged to drink alcohol by health professionals.

That these beliefs continue to be ingrained in current-day medical practice is evident from the findings of our recent study. We surveyed 410 lactating women living in the Delaware Valley about the type of advice, if any, they received about alcohol use during pregnancy and lactation. Approximately 25% of the women reported that a health professional (e.g., lactation consultant, midwife, physician, nurse) encouraged them to drink alcohol to improve the quality and quantity of their milk, to facilitate milk letdown, or to help their babies get a good night's sleep. This percentage is remarkably similar to that reported in the late 1970s (Dowdell, 1981). Approximately half of the women (54%) reported receiving no advice at all about alcohol use during lactation, whereas 21% were advised to refrain from drinking. A similar pattern emerged when we assessed the type of advice given by family members and friends (i.e., 19% were encouraged to drink, 69% received no advice at all, and 12% were discouraged from drinking).

The above finding is in striking contrast to the type of advice given to these women while they were pregnant. That is, the majority (55%) reported that they were advised by health professionals to abstain from drinking during pregnancy, whereas the remaining either received no advice at all (26%) or were advised to drink in moderation (19%). Thirteen women were encouraged to drink during the last trimester either to prevent miscarriages or because they were told that the baby would not be affected by alcohol at this late stage in fetal development. Of particular interest is the finding that 23% of the women whose health professionals had discouraged them from drinking alcohol while they were pregnant were encouraged to drink while they were lactating.

One of the reasons why such folklore persists may be the striking paucity of research on lactating women. The lack of scientific interest in alcohol consumption during lactation parallels an apparent lack of public concern. Epidemiological studies conducted in the 1980s revealed that although alcohol consumption decreased sharply after conception, it was not altered by the lactational status of the woman (Little, et al, 1990). Although women were less likely to smoke cigarettes or marijuana or to use cocaine if they elected to breastfeed, their 'regular' drinking patterns at one and three months postpartum were not significantly different from those women who never breastfed their infants, although they were less likely to report occasional binges of heavy drinking. Approximately 10% of the lactating women studied reported having at least one drink daily. Whether these women were drinking in response to the folklore is not known, but a recent study indicated that lactating women who were either encouraged to drink or who received no advice at all about alcohol reported drinking significantly more alcohol when compared to women who were advised not to drink (Mennella, 1997). To be sure, it is not known whether these women actually drank more or were more likely to admit they drank alcohol when compared to women who were discouraged to drink, or vice versa. Nevertheless, Blume (1987) has eloquently argued that health professionals should always be wary about prescribing alcohol as a drug to their patients for any indication since iatrogenic cases of alcoholism have been reported.

The Science of Alcohol Ingestion during Pregnancy and Lactation

What has the science, albeit limited, revealed to us about this folklore? The scientific investigation on the transfer of alcohol to human milk dates from the late 1890s. Maurice Nicloux, of the General Physiology Laboratories of the

Natural History Museum and the Tarnier Birth Clinic in Paris, demonstrated that the alcohol consumed by pregnant women could be detected in fetal blood (Nicloux, 1899a). After conducting an experiment on a lactating dog, Nicloux sought to determine whether the passage of alcohol also transferred to human milk. He collected milk samples before and at fixed intervals after wet nurses consumed 60 ml of a "Todd potion," which contained rum (45% alcohol), milk (120 ml), and sugar syrup (20 ml). The ethanol content in milk, which was almost identical to that detected in the woman's blood, peaked a half hour to one hour after ingestion and declined thereafter (Nicloux, 1899b; 1900).

These findings were replicated in several laboratories almost a century later (Kesaniemi, 1974; Lawton, 1985; Mennella and Beauchamp, 1991, 1993). We now know that the amount of alcohol transmitted to human milk is less than two percent of the maternal dose. However, there are considerable individual differences in the timing of peak levels and elimination rates in both milk and plasma. It is important to emphasize that by drinking alcohol shortly *before* breastfeeding, as recommended by the folklore, the mother optimizes the likelihood that the infant will be exposed to the alcohol in her milk.

The Science of Long-Term Effects of Postnatal Exposure to Alcohol

Despite the folklore, there is no controlled scientific evidence that supports the claim that

By drinking alcohol shortly before *breastfeeding, as recommended by the folklore, the mother optimizes the likelihood that the infant will be exposed to the alcohol in her milk.*

alcohol is a galactagogue. On the contrary, research findings have demonstrated that human infants consumed approximately 20% *less* breastmilk during the immediate hours following their mothers' consumption of an acute dose of alcohol (Mennella and Beauchamp, 1991, 1993), a finding that is consistent with several animal model studies (Subramanian and Abel, 1988; Swiatek, et al, 1986; Vilaro, et al, 1987). The observed decrease in milk intake was not the result of infants feeding for shorter time periods following maternal alcohol consumption (Mennella and Beauchamp, 1991, 1993). Nor was it related to infants rejecting the altered flavor in their mothers' milk, which also resulted from maternal alcohol consumption (Mennella, 1997). Rather, maternal alcohol consumption slightly, but significantly, reduced the amount of milk produced without altering its caloric content (Mennella, 1998).

Interestingly, mothers were apparently unaware of these differences in their lactational performance or their infants' behaviors (Mennella and Beauchamp, 1993). Because milk intake and the rate of synthesis of human milk

Contrary to the folklore, scientific studies revealed that maternal drinking diminshed milk intake at the breast and disrupted the infants' sleep patterning.

vary from feed to feed, a difference of this magnitude may be difficult for women to perceive. Moreover, it is often the infant, not the mother, who controls the pace and duration of breast-feeding and regulates milk intake. Perhaps one reason why the folklore that alcohol consumption (as well as other galactagogues) enhances lactational performance persisted for centuries, is because the breast-feeding mother does not have an immediate means of assessing how much milk her infant has consumed. In contrast, the bottle-feeding caretaker often feeds in response to the amount of formula remaining in the bottle. In other words, lactating women may be particularly susceptible to this type of folklore because of the many advantages that breastfeeding imparts on the infant.

Also, contrary to the folklore, maternal drinking disrupts the infants' sleep-wake patterning (Mennella and Gerrish, 1998). Infants, whose mothers drank little during both pregnancy and lactation, slept for significantly shorter periods during the 3.5 hours following the consumption of alcohol in their mothers' milk when compared to mothers' milk alone. This reduction was related, in part, to a shortening in the amount of time that the infants spent in active sleep, a finding consistent with that observed in the near-term fetus (Mulder, et al, 1998) and adults (Rundell, et al, 1972; Williams, et al, 1983).

Much less is known about the long-term effects of postnatal exposure to alcohol. In the only long-term study of the effects of lactational alcohol exposure in humans, Little and colleagues (1989) demonstrated that gross motor development at one year of age was slightly, but statistically significantly, altered in infants who were exposed regularly (at least daily) to alcohol in their mothers' milk. The association between maternal drinking and motor development persisted even after more than one hundred potentially confounding variables, including maternal tobacco, marijuana, and heavy caffeine use, were controlled for during pregnancy and the first three months after delivery. Moreover, the deficits in motor functioning were not attributable to alterations in maternal behaviors since infants whose mothers drank heavily (at least two drinks daily or engaged in binge drinking) but were weaned early, had significantly higher scores on motor development than did infants of heavy drinkers who were weaned at an older age (Little, et al, 1990). Rather, the deficits in motor develop-

Pumping the breasts and then discarding the milk does not hasten the disappearance of alcohol from breastmilk.

ment were most likely due to chronic exposure to alcohol in mothers' milk.

What Should We Recommend?

Based on these data, it would seem that the recommendation for a breastfeeding mother to drink a glass of beer or wine before nursing may be counterproductive. While mothers may be more relaxed after a drink, their babies will ingest less milk and their sleep will be disrupted. At the other extreme, it is not known how many women stop breastfeeding because of a concern about alcohol in their breastmilk. We do not want "science" to frighten women. Unlike that which occurs during pregnancy, women who drink occasionally during lactation can limit their infants' exposure to alcohol by timing breastfeeds in relation to drinking. And, contrary to popular beliefs, alcohol is not stored in breastmilk but parallels that found in maternal plasma, peaking approximately 30-60 minutes after drinking and decreasing thereafter. In other words, pumping the breast and then discarding the milk does not hasten the disappearance of alcohol from the milk.

The goal of our research program is to experimentally investigate the relationship between alcohol and breastfeeding so that we can provide mothers and health professionals with some answers to frequently asked questions on this topic. Now, when a nursing mothers is told that drinking alcohol will help her baby sleep better or gain weight, she and her caregivers can refer to the research that calls this lore into serious question.

References

Blume S (1987). Beer and the breast-feeding mom. *Journal of the American Medical Association* 258 (15), 2126.

Davidson S, Alden L, Davidson P (1981). Changes in alcohol consumption after childbirth. *Journal of Advanced Nursing* 6 (3), 195-98.

Dowdell PM (1981). Alcohol and pregnancy: A review of the literature 1968-1980. *Nursing Times* 77 (43), 1826-31.

Kesaniemi YI (1974). Ethanol and acetaldehyde in the milk and peripheral blood of lactating women after ethanol administration. *Journal of Obstetrics and Gynaecology of the British Commonwealth* 81, 84-86.

Krebs R (1953). *Making Friends is our Business— 100 years of Anheuser Busch*. Missouri: Anheuser Busch, Inc., pp.434-37.

Lawton ME (1985). Alcohol in breast milk. *Australian Journal of Obstetrics and Gynaecology* 25 (1),71-73.

Little RE (1990). Maternal use of alcohol and breast-fed infants—reply. *New England Journal of Medicine* 322 (5), 339.

Little RE, Anderson KW, Ervin CH, Worthington-Roberts B, Clarren SK (1989). Maternal alcohol use during breast feeding and infant mental and motor development at one year. *New England Journal of Medicine* 321 (7), 425-30.

Little RE, Lambert MD, Worthington-Roberts B (1990). Drinking and smoking at 3 months postpartum by lactation history. *Paediatrics and Perinatal Epidemiology* 4 (3), 290-302.

Mennella JA (1998). Short-term effects of maternal alcohol consumption on lactational performance. *Alcoholism: Clinical and Experimental Research* 22 (7):1389-92.

Mennella JA (1997). The human infants' suckling responses to the flavor of alcohol in mothers' milk. *Alcoholism: Clinical and Experimental Research* 21 (4), 581-85.

Mennella JA, Beauchamp GK (1991). The transfer of alcohol to human milk: Effects on flavor and the infant's behavior. *New England Journal of Medicine* 325 (14), 981-85.

Mennella JA, Beauchamp GK (1993). Beer, breast feeding and folklore. *Developmental Psychobiology* 26 (8), 459-66.

Mennella JA, Gerrish CJ (1998). Effects of exposure to alcohol in mother's milk on infant sleep. *Pediatrics* 101 (5): e21-25.

Mulder EJH, Morssink LP, Van Der Schee T, Visser GHA (1998). Acute maternal alcohol consumption disrupts behavioral state organization in the near-term fetus. *Pediatric Research* 44 (5), 774-79.

Nicloux M (1899a). Sur le passage de l'alcool ingere de la mere au foetus, en particulier chez la femme. *Comptes Rendus de la Societe de Biologie, Paris* 6, 980-82.

Nicloux M (1899b). Sur le passage de l'alcool ingere de la lait chez la femme. *Comptes Rendus de la Societe de Biologie, Paris* 6, 982-84.

Nicloux M (1900). Dosage comparatif de l'alcool dans le sang de la mere et du foetus et dans le lait apres ingestion d'alcool : Remarquees sur le dosage de l'alcool dans le sang et dans le lait. *Comptes Rendus Academie des Sciences* 80, 855-58.

Robinovitch LG (1903). Infantile alcoholism. *Quarterly Journal of Inebriety* 25, 231-36.

Routh CHF (1879). *Infant Feeding and its Influence on Life.* New York: William Wood and Company; pp. 71-87.

Rundell OH, Lester BK, Griffiths WJ, Williams HL (1972). Alcohol and sleep in young adults. *Psychopharmacologia (Berlin)* 26 (3), 201-18.

Subramanian MG, Abel EL (1988). Alcohol inhibits suckling-induced prolactin release and milk yield. *Alcohol* 5 (2), 95-98.

Swiatek KR, Dombrowski, Jr. GJ, Chao K-L (1986). The inefficient transfer of maternally fed alcohol to nursing rats. *Alcohol* 3 (3), 169-74.

Vilaro S, Vinas O, Remesar X, Herrera E (1987). Effects of chronic ethanol consumption on lactational performance in the rat: Mammary gland and milk composition and pups' growth and metabolism. *Pharmacology Biochemistry and Behavior* 27 (2), 333-39.

Williams DL, MacLean AW, Cairns J (1983). Dose-response effects of ethanol on the sleep of young women. *Journal of Studies on Alcohol* 44 (3), 515-23.

Articles

Feeding Patterns of Preterm Infants post NICU Discharge

Sharon Piper, PhD, RN, MPH

Sharon Piper is Assistant Professor, Catholic University of America, School of Nursing, Washington, DC. This study was funded by a Faculty Grant-in-Aid, Catholic University of America. These data were initially presented at the Annual ILCA Conference, July 2000. Contact the author at the School of Nursing, Catholic University of America, Gowan Hall, Washington, DC 20064 USA.

Current Issues in Clinical Lactation, 2002, 11–21; breastfeeding, feeding patterns, human lactation, preterm infants, NICU.

Abstract

This study examines the intensity of breastmilk exposure for a convenience sample of premature infants over ten weeks after discharge from the neonatal intensive care unit (NICU). A non-experimental, descriptive, longitudinal design was used. Calculated as a ratio of breastmilk feeds to all liquid feeds, the average intensity of breastmilk exposure ranged from 0.19 at discharge to 0.372 two weeks after discharge. There was a significant difference in average levels of intensity across the ten-week period (Wilks lambda $= 0.756$, $F = 4.309$, $(3, 40)$ $p = 0.01$). High intensity was significantly associated with a vaginal delivery, high intensity at day of discharge from the NICU, and the mother's longer intended duration of breastfeeding.

Introduction

There is limited information in the breastfeeding literature about the feeding patterns of premature infants after they are discharged from the NICU (Meier, 1997). Characteristics of preterm infants who breastfed while in the NICU include a higher birthweight, decreased need for oxygen and ventilator support, and the absence of bottle-feeding (Hedberg Nyqvist and Ewald, 1999). For most preterm infants, however, the NICU feeding experience includes a variety of nutritional sources (at the breast, expressed breastmilk from a bottle, formula in a bottle, oral-gastric [OG] or naso-gastric [NG] feedings) (Meier, et al, 1993). It is not known if this pattern of varied feedings continues after discharge, or if feeding at the breast eventually becomes the primary feeding pattern as the infant matures. Maternal concerns about the adequacy of their premature infant's milk intake post discharge led to identifying a "turning point" in the breastfeeding of premature infants at home after discharge. Kavanaugh, et al (1995) identified this turning point as occurring approximately two weeks after discharge when infant weight gain, indicators of satiety, and longer duration of feeding episodes (among other factors) indicated to the mothers that their infants were "getting enough." This turning point appeared to coincide with the infants achieving approximately 38 weeks post-conceptual age. What is not known is if supplementary bottle-feeds (to insure adequate milk intake) declined after this turning point, leading to an increase in the intensity of breastfeeding.

Assessment of feeding patterns provides information on exposure to breastmilk. Level of breastmilk exposure determines the "biologic potency" of breastfeeding, with the assumption that an increasing level of exposure to breastmilk increases its prophylactic (protective) effect with respect to infection and other illnesses (Kramer, 1988). The growing preterm infant in the NICU will experience greater nutritional needs to support growth and development than at any other point in its life span. Presumably, the longer a preterm infant only receives breastmilk (rather than other nutrients) the greater its protective effect (Schanler and Atkinson, 1999; Garza, Butte, and Goldman, 1993; Kramer, 1988). This is particularly relevant as premature infants may be more vulnerable to health threats such as infections and atopic illnesses and would be likely to benefit from greater intensity of exposure to breastmilk (Scariati, et al, 1997; Ford and Labbok, 1993; Cunningham, Jelliffe, and Jelliffe, 1991).

Purpose

The purpose of this study was to examine and describe the feeding patterns of premature infants within the first ten weeks after their discharge from the NICU. Specifically, the study was designed to examine the intensity of breastmilk exposure (that, is, the ratio of breastmilk feeds to all liquid feeds received) for the premature infant. Maternal concerns about the adequacy of their premature infant's intake of breastmilk are presumed to lead to a mother's

The purpose of this study is to examine and describe one aspect of the premature infant's experience; specifically, feeding patterns within the first ten weeks after discharge from the NICU.

increased supplementation with formula. Such supplementation may also lead to premature weaning from the breast. An examination of the intensity of exposure to breastmilk in the premature population provides information about initial patterns of breastfeeding and supplementation, as well as whether breastfeeding increases or declines in practice as the infant matures and grows.

Research Questions

The following research questions were addressed:

1) What are the feeding patterns of premature infants at discharge and at two, six, and ten weeks after discharge?

2) What is the level of breastfeeding intensity at discharge and at two, six, and ten weeks after discharge?

3) Does the level of breastfeeding intensity change over time within ten weeks after discharge?

4) What factors are associated with breastfeeding intensity over time within ten weeks after discharge?

Variable of Interest

Intensity of exposure to breastmilk is conceptualized as the ratio of the number of breastmilk feeds to total liquid feeds received (Piper SL, *Duration and intensity of breastfeeding as predictors of child health status after weaning.* Unpublished doctoral dissertation, University of Maryland, Baltimore; 1996). It is operationalized as the number of feeds at the breast, plus the number of expressed breastmilk (EBM) feeds divided by the total number of feeds at the breast, plus the number of EBM feeds, plus the number of formula feeds at a given point in time. This calculation provides a ratio with a range between 0.0 and 1.0 The closer the ratio is to 1.0, the higher the level of intensity of exposure to breastmilk. This ratio can easily be incorporated into the Interagency Group for Action on Breastfeeding (IGAB) schema and framework of breastfeeding definitions (Labbok and Krasovec, 1990). For this study, a calculation of the intensity ratio for a given subject was as follows: data on feeding patterns (number of feeds at the breast, number of EBM feeds, and number of formula feeds) were collected daily for a week at a time using seven-day feeding diaries. Intensity levels were calculated for each of the seven days, and a mean was calculated for each specific week. As demonstrated, the intensity ratio may be calculated for a specific period or over a time period deemed relevant for clinical or research purposes.

Methods

Research Design and Sample. This study was a non-experimental, descriptive, comparative study with data collected longitudinally. This non-probability sample included 43 mothers and their premature infants, who were admitted to the NICU of a full-service suburban teaching hospital in the eastern United States over a six-month period. Lactation services at these institutions were provided at an off-site lactation center and through daily post-delivery lactation rounds on the maternal-newborn unit during the study period. Over the six-month period of subject enrollment, 48 newborns met the inclusion criteria. Inclusion criteria specified that the infant was between 30 and 36 weeks assessed gestational age at the time of delivery; the infant had no congenital anomalies that would impede breastfeeding; the mothers planned to breastfeed the infant prior to and after discharge from the hospital; the mothers were 18 years of age or older; and, the mothers could read, write, and speak English sufficiently to complete the interview and the feeding diaries. Five mothers declined participation in the study. The sample size of 43 provided sufficient power (0.831) to conduct the repeated measure one-way analysis of variance used to answer the research questions.

Measures/Instruments

The principal investigator developed instruments used to collect the data. Content validity of the tools was ascertained in consultation with two nurse experts, one of whom was a lactation consultant, and the other a nurse-researcher in maternal-child health. The instruments used to collect data included a demographic and pregnancy history survey, a day of discharge feeding survey, and a seven-day feeding diary. Mothers were first interviewed (for demographic and pregnancy history) within 24-48 hours after delivery after receiving an explanation of the study and giving informed consent. Feeding pattern data were collected from the mothers on the day of their infant's discharge from the NICU (day of discharge feeding survey), and at two, six, and ten weeks after discharge, using the seven-day feeding diaries. Data relating to the delivery and specifics of the infant's stay in the NICU were collected using a medical charge survey. Reliability of the feeding diary data—used to calculate the intensity ratio—was strengthened by the calculation of mean intensity ratios over seven days' time. In addition, during the second, sixth, and tenth weeks after discharge, daily intensity ratios were not significantly different, indicating consistency of feeding pattern data over a given weekly period.

Data Analysis

Exploratory data analysis was conducted, and descriptive statistics appropriate to the level of measure were used to describe the sample on all variables. To address research questions 1 and 2, intensity ratios were calculated for day of discharge and two, six, and ten weeks after discharge. Frequencies of these ratios were determined based on the schema and framework categories of full and partial breastfeeding (Labbok and Krasovec, 1990), and average intensity ratios were calculated for each time period. To address research question 3, which compares average levels of intensity over time, a within-subjects (repeated measures) one-way analysis of variance (ANOVA) with post-hoc testing was calculated. Research question 4 was addressed by examining correlations between variables using Pearson's r and Spearman rho. Alpha was set at 0.05 for all analyses.

Findings

Newborns. Average gestational age by assessment at time of delivery was 33.9 weeks. The mean birth weight for the sample was 2206 gms, and mean weight on day of discharge was 2314 gm, although at discharge 29 of the infants (69%) weighed more than 2500 gms. The majority of the babies were male (58%), and their average length of stay in the NICU was 14.7 days (range: 1-48 days). Fourteen newborns (33%) received ventilatory support in the NICU, 34 (79%) received IV fluids, and 24 (56%) received NG or OG feedings. For 27 (63%) of the infants, the 5-minute APGAR score was 9.

Mothers. Average age of the mothers was 32 years. Twenty-two mothers (51%) were non-Hispanic Caucasian, 13 (30%) were African American, four (9%) were Asian, three (7%) were East Indian, and one mother identified herself as Hispanic. Sixteen mothers (37%) had completed college, and 11 mothers (26%) reported an educational level beyond college. Most mothers (86%) were married to the baby's father, and 81% of the women reported that they were employed and would be returning to work. Twenty-nine mothers (67%) delivered vaginally. Seventeen mothers were primiparas (40%); however, for nearly as many (15; 35%) their preterm infant was at least their third child. For most, this was their first preterm birth; for nine women (21%), this was their second preterm birth. Maternal complications were the reason for 31 (72%) of the preterm deliveries, although only 3 of the women (7%) spent any time prior to delivery in the high-risk antepartum unit.

Breastfeeding. The decision to breastfeed was made prior to their pregnancy for 30 (70%) of the mothers; 29 women (67%) were breastfeeding for the first time. Twenty-four of the mothers (56%) planned to breastfeed fully after their infants came home; average planned duration of breastfeeding was 218 days (7 months) (median: 210 days; mode: 1 year). Most of the women (34; 79%) had obtained an electric breast pump for home use through the lactation center, and most began pumping one day after the baby's preterm birth. On the day of discharge from the NICU, 28 mothers (65%) reported that they had frozen breastmilk at home, and 39 (91%) reported having breast-fed their baby in the NICU. At discharge, 38 (88%) of the mothers reported that they felt comfortable with their ability to feed the infant at home either at the breast or with formula.

Feeding patterns and level of intensity over time. Table 1 shows the frequency of the intensity ratios based on the IAGB schema and framework for breastfeeding definitions (Labbok and Krasovec, 1990). Changes in the frequency of intensity occur-red over the ten weeks after discharge, with the frequency of any breastfeeding behavior decreasing over time. Full breast-feeding increased in frequency from day of discharge to two weeks after discharge. During this time, the frequency of high partial breastfeeding also increased. These changes are consistent with the "turning point" described at two weeks after discharge (Kavanaugh, et al, 1995) and are accompanied by a decrease in the frequency of medium and low partial feeding patterns. At six weeks post discharge, high partial and medium partial feeding patterns had begun to decline in frequency, with a subsequent increase in low partial breastfeeding and weaning behaviors. Full breastfeeding declined at six weeks to previous day of discharge levels but increased again at ten weeks post discharge. These changes in frequency over time are further illustrated by the variation in average level of intensity over the four time periods (See Table 1). Average intensity of breastmilk exposure ranged from 0.19 at day of discharge to 0.372 at two weeks after discharge. Mean intensity at six weeks (0.304) and ten weeks (0.235) after discharge declined from this peak (see Table 2).

Comparison of average intensity over time. A within-subjects (repeated measures) ANOVA was performed to compare average intensity levels across time periods. In addition, repeated measures ANOVA were used to compare daily

Table 1. Frequency of Intensity of Exposure to Breastmilk Levels Over Time (N = 43).

	Breastmilk Levels								
	Full		High		Medium		Low		No	
	f	(%)	f	(%)	f	(%)	f	(%)	f	(%)
Day of discharge	1	(2)	0	(—)	14	(23)	10	(23)	18	(42)
2 wks post discharge	4	(9)	8	(18)	11	(25)	1	(2)	19	(44)
6 wks post discharge	1	(2)	8	(18)	8	(18)	3	(7)	23	(54)
10 wks post discharge	2	(5)	5	(12)	6	(14)	1	(2)	29	(67)

a Intensity ratio = 1.0
b Intensity ratio = ≤1.0 and ≥.80
c Intensity ratio = ≥.21 to ≤.79
d Intensity ratio = ≤.20
e Intensity ratio = 0

Table 2. Average Intensity of Exposure to Breastmilk Levels for Four Time Periods (N = 43)

Time	Mean	Median	Mode	SD
Day of discharge	.1905	.111	.00	.2312
Two wks post discharge	.3717	.2168	.00	.4030
Six wks post discharge	.3036	.000	.00	.3921
Ten wks post discharge	.2347	.000	.00	.3759

intensity levels within each week of data collection. This test assumes that difference scores are multivariately normally distributed in the population, and that scores are independent of each other between subjects (Green, Salkind and Akey, 1999). A significant difference in average levels of intensity over time (day of discharge and two, six, and ten weeks after discharge) was found (see Table 3). Post-hoc testing using pair-wise comparisons with a bonferroni corrected level of alpha (<.008; 6 sixomparison/.05) indicated a significant difference in intensity between day of discharge and two weeks after discharge (t = 3.492, df = 42, p = .001, two-tailed test). During the second, sixth, and tenth weeks after discharge, daily intensity levels were not found to be significantly different, indicating consistency of feeding patterns over a given week (see Table 3).

Variables associated with intensity of breastfeeding. Table 4 documents the significant correlates to intensity of breastmilk exposure over time. What is most noteworthy is the statistically significant relationships between levels of intensity over time. A higher level of intensity at each time period is associated with a higher level of intensity at the subsequent time period. When average intensity levels at subsequent periods are examined, this pattern is maintained. These findings are consistent with associations found among intensity levels over six months in a national sample (Piper SL. *Duration and intensity of breastfeeding as predictors of child health status after weaning.* Unpublished doctoral dissertation, University of Maryland, Baltimore, 1996). Planned duration of breastfeeding also demonstrated moderate to strong associations with higher level of intensity at two, six, and ten weeks after discharge, as did the timing of a mother's decision to breastfeed her baby. A mother's pre-pregnancy decision to breastfeed was associated with a higher level of intensity at six and ten weeks after discharge. A vaginal birth was also associated with higher levels of intensity at two, six, and ten weeks after discharge. Higher level of maternal education was associated with higher intensity at 10 weeks post discharge; the infant's greater gestational age was associated with higher intensity at six weeks after discharge; and, maternal gravidity, no previous preterm deliveries, and prior experience breastfeeding were associated with higher intensity at two weeks after discharge. Timing of postpartum return to employment (in weeks postpartum) and race were not associated with average intensity levels at any time period.

Table 3. Repeated Measures ANOVA – Comparison of Intensity of Exposure to Breastmilk Levels Over Ten Weeks Post NICU Discharge (N = 43)

	Value	F	Df	Statistical Significance	Eta squared
Wilks Lambda	.756	4.309	3,40	0.01	.244

Repeated Measures ANOVA – Comparison of Intensity of Exposure to Breastmilk Levels over Seven Days at 2, 6, and 10 weeks post NICU Discharge.

	Value	F	Df	Statistical Significance	Eta squared
At 2 wks Wilks Lambda	.859	1.010	6,37	.437	.141
At 6 wks Wilks Lambda	.870	.925	6,37	.488	.130
At 10 wks Wilks Lambda	.845	1.127	6,37	.366	.155

Conclusions

This sample of preterm newborns demonstrated variable patterns of feeding over ten weeks after their discharge from the NICU. Supplementary feedings increased over time, formula became the predominant feeding choice, and at ten weeks after discharge, 29 (67%) of the sample had completely weaned from breastfeeding. The benchmarks for breastfeeding duration identified by Healthy People 2010 goals and AAP recommendations are not met for the majority of this sample (USDHHS, 2000; AAP, 1997). Nevertheless, the findings demonstrate a statistically significant change in level of intensity between day of discharge and two weeks after discharge. During this time period, the level of intensity increased by almost 20 percentage points. This increase in the average level of intensity supports the findings of Kavanaugh, et al (1995) who found that mothers identified a feeding "turning point" approximately two weeks after discharge, at about 38 weeks gestational age. Based on this sample's average gestational age of 33.9 weeks, and average length of stay in the NICU of 14.9 days, these newborns were approximately 38 weeks gestation at the time of demonstrated statistically significant increase in breastfeeding intensity two weeks after discharge. While gestational age at discharge can only be estimated within this data set, these findings provide further support for a turning point when breastmilk intake and breastfeeding behaviors increase. Higher levels of intensity at two weeks post discharge are

Table 4. Corelates with Intensity of Exposure to Breastmilk Levels Over Three Post Discharge Time Periods (N=43)

	2 wks	6 wks	10 wks
Age of youngest child(years)	.356*		
Average intensity, 2 wks post discharge		.807**	.583**
Average intensity, 6 wks post discharge		.759**	
Intensity, day of discharge	.537**	.500**	.307**
Time of decision to breastfeed baby		−.333*#	−.442**#
Type of delivery+	−.333*#	−.348*#	−.399**#
First time breastfeeding++	.306*#		
Gestational age at delivery (weeks)	.324*		
Mothers' years of education (years)			.431**
Maternal gravida status	.342*		
Number, previous preterm deliveries	−.334*		
Planned duration of breastfeeding (days)	.380*	.549**	.619**
Longest duration of breastfeeding (days)	.315*		

* alpha = .05
** alpha = .01
# Spearman rho, all other correlations Pearson's r
^ prior to pregnancy = 1, during pregnancy = 2, after delivery = 3
+ vaginal = 1, cesarean = 2
++ yes = 1, no = 2

A higher level of intensity at each time period is associated with a higher level of intensity at the subsequent time period.

associated with higher levels of intensity at six and ten weeks after discharge; however, a majority of the sample (54%) had weaned by six weeks after discharge. The declines in the average level of intensity between two and six weeks, and six and ten weeks after discharge

are not statistically significant, but they do have implications for clinical practice. For this sample, decreased average level of intensity cannot be explained by timing of return to employment by the mothers.

Implications for Practice

When examining the implications for practice within the context of a research study, it is important to look at the factors that may be influenced by clinical practice found to be associated with desirable outcomes. The associations found between intensity at day of discharge and intensity levels in subsequent weeks, as well as the associations between other variables, have implications for clinical practice because these factors may be influenced by clinicians. The timing of a woman's decision to breastfeed a future child, as well as the length of time she plans to breastfeed that child may be influenced by culturally appropriate pre-pregnancy and prenatal education for well women and pregnant women. Intensity of breastmilk exposure at day of discharge from the NICU may potentially be influenced by the clinician's consistent and rigorous efforts directed toward maximizing feeds at the breast as well as feeds with expressed breastmilk while the newborn is in the NICU. Increasing levels of intensity of breastmilk exposure at two weeks after discharge and beyond may by influenced by frequent, periodic support and contact with a lactation professional to facilitate achievement of the mother's original (or revised) breastfeeding goals. The use of a non-probability sample of this study prevents gener-alizing beyond this sample to feeding patterns after discharge from the NICU in other settings. Nevertheless, these findings are consistent with what is known about the preterm newborn and breastfeeding, and they provide further evidence of the need for clinicians to support the mother in her efforts to provide her preterm infant with access to the breast and to breast-milk, both prior to discharge and during the critical first ten weeks at home.

References

American Academy of Pediatrics Work Group on Breastfeeding (1997). Breastfeeding and the use of human milk. *Pediatrics* 100 (6), 1035-39.

Cunningham AS, Jelliffe DB, Jelliffe EFP (1991). Breastfeeding and health in the 1980s: A global epidemiological review. *Journal of Pediatrics* 118 (5), 659-66.

Ford K, Labbok M (1993). Breastfeeding and child health in the United States. *Journal of Biosocial Science* 25, 187-94.

Garza C, Butte NF, Goldman AS (1993). Human milk and infant formula. In: Suskind RM, and Lewinter-Suskind L, Eds. *Textbook of Pediatric Nutrition*, 2nd ed. New York: Raven Press, pp. 33-42.

Green SB, Salkind NJ, Akey TM (1999). *Using SPSS for Windows: Analyzing and Understanding Data*. New Jersey: Prentice-Hall, pp. 251-62.

Hedberg Nyqvist K, Ewald U (1999). Infant and maternal factors in the development of breastfeeding behavior and breastfeeding outcome in preterm infants. *Acta Paediatrica* 88 (11), 1194-1203.

Intensity of breastmilk exposure at day of discharge may potentially be influenced by the clinician's consistent and rigorous efforts directed towards maximizing feeds at the breast as well as feeds with expressed breastmilk while the newborn is in the NICU.

Kavanaugh K, Mead L, Meier P, Mangurten HH (1995). Getting enough: Mothers' concerns about breastfeeding a premature infant after discharge. *Journal of Obstetric, Gynecologic, and Neonatal Nursing* 24 (1), 23-32.

Kramer MS (1988). Does breastfeeding help protect against atopic disease? Biology, methodology, and a golden jubilee of controversy. *Journal of Pediatrics* 112 (2), 181-90.

Labbok MH, Krasovec K (1990). Towards consistency in breastfeeding definitions. *Studies in Familiy Planning* 21 (4), 226-30.

Meier PP (1997). *Professional Guide to Breastfeeding Premature Infants*. Columbus, Ohio: Ross Products Division, Abbott Laboratories; pp.1-3.

Meier PP, Engstrom JL, Mangurten HH, Estrada E, Zimmerman B, Kopparthi R (1993). Breastfeeding support services in the neonatal intensive care unit. *Journal of Obstetric, Gynecologic, and Neonatal Nursing* 22 (4), 338-47.

Scariati PD, Grummer-Strawn LM, Fein SB (1997). A longitudinal analysis of infant morbidity and the extent of breastfeeding in the United States. *Pediatrics* 99 (6), e1-5.

Schanler RJ, Atkinson SA (1999). Effects of nutrients in human milk on the recipient premature infant. *Journal of Mammary Gland Biology and Neoplasia* 4 (3), 297-307.

USDHHS (2000). *Healthy People 2010: Conference Edition*. US Government Printing Office: Washington, DC, pp.16-48.

A Comparison of Long-term Breastfeeding Among Hispanics and Non-Hispanics

Kathleen M. Buckley, PhD, RN, IBCLC

Kathleen Buckley is an Assistant Professor in the School of Nursing at Catholic University of America. This research was supported by an individual National Research Service Award (No. 1 F31 NR06678-01) from the Department of Health and Human Services of the US Public Health Service. Contact the author at Catholic University of America, School of Nursing, 620 Michigan Avenue NE, Washington, DC 20064 USA.

Current Issues in Clinical Lactation, 2002, 23–35; extended breastfeeding, Hispanic, infant feeding practices, long-term breastfeeding, social support.

Abstract

This study examines maternal beliefs and practices associated with long-term breastfeeding beyond infancy. The sample includes 40 mothers (10 Hispanics and 30 non-Hispanics) who lived in a metropolitan area. Semi-structured interviews occurred in the mother's home. Both groups emphasized breastfeeding as a natural choice promoting mother-child attachment. Differences among the two groups included their initial exposure to extended breastfeeding, the decision to engage and continue breastfeeding past their child's first birthday, the degree of their concealment of continued breastfeeding, and sources of support. Health professionals need to recognize why mothers of different ethnic groups in the United States choose to maintain long-term breastfeeding by providing support for a practice reported to be associated with a negative social stigma.

Introduction

Human milk is optimally adapted to meet the nutritional requirements and physiological needs of the infant in all societies. Breastfeeding confers nutritional and immunologic advantages for the child, as well as health, economic, contraceptive, and psychosocial advantages for the mother. On the basis of these findings, a U.S. national breastfeeding goal established as part of the Healthy People 2000 initiative was to increase to at least 50 percent the proportion of mothers who breastfeed until their infants are five to six months old (U.S. Dept. of Health and Human Services, 1990). The American Academy of Pediatrics recommends that breastfeeding continue for at least a year, and longer as mutually desired (AAP, 1997). On an international level, the World Health Organization advocates breastfeeding for the first two years or more (UNICEF/WHO, 1990). Beyond a year of age, breastmilk has been found to be a useful additional source of nutrients for children (Dewey, Finley, & Lönnerdal, 1984) and a continuing source of protective immunities (Lawrence, 1994).

In a retrospective study of U.S. and Canadian mothers' perceptions of the consequences of long-term breastfeeding, Kendall-Tackett and Sugarman (1995) identify the "social stigma" associated with the practice. Mothers cite this negative aspect of continuing to breast-feed as increasing as the child ages. In some cases, mothers engaged in extended breastfeeding have been accused of sexually abusing their children (Wilson-Clay, 1990). In response to perceived disapproval of extended breastfeeding in the U.S., mothers who nurse the older infant/child often practice some form of "closet nursing"; that is, breastfeeding carried out with some degree of secrecy (Avery, 1977). Mothers may also encourage the use of a "code word" by their child for breastfeeding.

Differences in meanings and practices among the two groups included (1) the initial exposure and decision to engage in extended breastfeeding; (2) reasons for continuing to breastfeed past their child's first birthday; (3) the degree of concealment of the practice; and, (4) the mothers' primary sources of social support.

A large national mail survey reports low breastfeeding rates at 12 months of age, specifically 16.8 percent among Hispanics, 14.7 percent among Whites, and 9.9 percent among Black women (Ross Mothers' Surveys. Updated breastfeeding trend through 1997. Unpublished raw data.) The prevalence of breastfeeding beyond a year of age is not clear.

While some cultural research in the U.S. of middle income, White mothers who practice extended breastfeeding is reported (Bottorff,

1990; Buckley, 1992; Wrigley & Hutchinson, 1990), there is little information on mothers' motivations and practices in continuing to breastfeed the older child in the United States among different ethnic groups.

This study sought to examine the reasons non-Hispanic and Hispanic mothers give for continuing to breastfeed a child beyond a year of age and to identify any differences in the practice among the two ethnic groups and their primary sources of support for the practice.

Methods

Design. This study used an exploratory/descriptive design (Nieswiadomy, 1998) to uncover some of the underlying meanings and practices associated with long-term breastfeeding (defined as breastfeeding a child past the first year birthday) in two ethnic groups (Hispanic and non-Hispanic) in a major U.S. metropolitan area. After obtaining written informed consent, data on mothers' reasons for practicing extended breastfeeding were collected through home interviews by the principal investigator. Sixty-eight open-ended questions were included in at least two intensive home interviews, each lasting one to two hours. Topics included influences on breastfeeding, practical considerations and challenges, and weaning, feeding and parenting practices. For example, under the category of "Influences on Breastfeeding," each mother was asked, "How did it happen that your child continued to breastfeed after a year of age?" and "Who or what influenced you the most to continue breastfeeding?"

The interview guide was developed in consultation with experts in the field of nutritional anthropology and child development, and was pilot tested with four mothers who were engaged in long-term breastfeeding. Their feedback regarding clarity of questions and suggestions for additional response options helped to establish face and content validity of the instrument.

Following each interview, mothers' tape recorded responses were transcribed verbatim and coded according to the type of question asked during the interview. A content analysis (Miles & Huberman, 1994) of the words used by the informant was followed by analysis of the questions, which involved reading transcribed interviews and noting repeated patterns and themes. Words used to describe similar concepts were clustered under an umbrella term, unless a specific word or phrase was used frequently by informants. Analyzed responses were also grouped by the mother's ethnicity. Finally, metaphors were developed in an effort to conceptualize mothers' meanings and practices related to long-term breastfeeding.

Sample. The sample included 40 mothers who lived in the Washington, D.C. metropolitan area who were practicing long-term breastfeeding. Due to the hidden nature and negative social stigma associated with extended breastfeeding, the participants were selected through purposive sampling. Subjects who were continuing to breastfeed a child past their first year birthday were recruited through contacts with local pediatricians, nurses working in community health centers, and La Leche League members. All of the women described themselves as Caucasian. Ten were Hispanic and emigrated to the United States from the Spanish speaking Caribbean islands or Central or South America (see Table 1). Thirty were non-Hispanic, were born in the United States, and were of European descent.

The Hispanic women had been residents of the United States for 1 to 23 years (mean length of stay was 9 years). All had arrived in the D.C. metropolitan area as a young adult (range: 18-30 years of age). Based on 1990 Census data, the Hispanic ethnic groups as identified by country of origin were similar to the current Hispanic population residing in the District of Columbia metropolitan area at the time of the study (U.S. Bureau of Census, 1995). Seven Hispanic mothers were fully fluent in English and Spanish; three others spoke only Spanish. A Spanish speaking interpreter was used at the time of the interviews to translate for the principal investigator the comments of these three

Table 1. Country of Origin of Hispanic Mothers

Country of Origin	Number of Subjects
El Salvador	3
Dominican Republic	2
Colombia	1
Guatemala	1
Nicaragua	1
Peru	1
Puerto Rico	1
TOTAL	10

mothers. The 30 non-Hispanic mothers were monolingual English speakers.

Mothers' ages ranged from 25 to 45 years and were similar across groups. The Hispanic mothers were younger, had fewer years of education, and more likely to be fulltime homemakers and to have a lower income than the non-Hispanic women (see Table 2). Forty-one children (25 boys and 16 girls) were breastfeeding. Although only 40 mothers were enrolled in the study, two of the White, non-Hispanic mothers were tandem breast-feeding non-twin siblings. One was breastfeeding two children each over a year of age, and the other a six-month-old infant and a child older than a year. The children's ages ranged from 12 to 44 months with no significant difference among groups.

Findings

Differences in meanings and practices between the two groups included their (1) initial exposure to extended breastfeeding and their decision to engage in extended breastfeeding, (2) reasons for continuing to breastfeed past the child's first year birthday, (3) the degree of concealment of the practice, and (4) the mothers' primary sources of social support (see Table 3).

Initial exposure. The Hispanic mothers were first exposed to long-term breastfeeding during their childhood. Although their Hispanic ethnicity varied, the mothers stated that breastfeeding children up to four years of age was common in their countries of origin. Many of the Hispanic mothers recalled seeing a member

Table 2. Demographic Characteristics of Breastfeeding Hispanic and Non-Hispanic Mothers

Characteristics	Hispanic Mothers	Non-Hispanic Mothers
Maternal Age (yrs)		
Range	25-45	27-41
Mode	31	37
Median	31	35
Mean	32	35
Child's Age (months)		
Range	13-44	12-42
Mode	3	15
Median	17.5	20
Mean	24.5	21.7
Maternal education (yrs)		
Range	4-18	13-20
Mode	4	18
Median	12.3	17.5
Mean	11.6	16.9
Maternal employment status		
Working for pay fulltime	0	1 (3%)
Working for pay part-time	2 (20%)	9 (30%)
Fulltime homemakers	8 (80%)	20 (67%)
Household size		
Range	3-7	3-6
Mode	4	4
Median	4	4
Mean	4.2	3.9
Household Annual Income ($K)		
Range	8.5-60	28-175
Mode	20	70
Median	20	60
Mean	25	65

of their family breastfeeding a child older than a year of age. When asked to describe their initial reaction, they stated that breastfeeding was a part of their daily living and a normal custom.

The Hispanic mothers' decision to continue

Table 3. Meanings and Practices of Extended Breastfeeding among Hispanic and non-Hispanic Mothers

Practice of extended breastfeeding	Hispanic mothers (N = 10)	Non-Hispanic mothers (N = 30)
Timing of and reaction to first exposure	occurred as a child with minimal reaction	occurred as an adult with shock and surprise
Decision to engage in extended breastfeeding	made prior to or shortly after birth	evolved slowly over the first year after birth through contact with other mothers engaged in the practice
Perception as "natural or normal thing to do"	a familiar custom in country of origin	based on a normal biological process of child feeding
Primary advantages	nutritional reasons, health maintenance	to nurture and comfort the child
Degree of secrecy	less familiarity with or interest in use of "closet nursing" or "code word" by the child	practiced "closet nursing" and promoted use of "code word" by the child

breastfeeding was often made prior to or shortly after the birth of their child and was based upon a custom with which they were familiar. One Hispanic mother stated, "My mother breastfed all her children until they were three and close to four. I knew about my grandmother doing that, and my aunts, then, my cousins. It has been what I grew up seeing."

In contrast, the non-Hispanic mothers described their first exposure to toddler breastfeeding as an eye-opening experience. They had no idea that this practice existed and was more common than they expected. Generally the non-Hispanic mothers' first reaction to extended breastfeeding was shock and aversion. Although many wanted to breastfeed, they initially believed they would never do it beyond a year. The following comment was typical:

I thought it was strange the first time I saw it. I thought, 'The kid looks so big.' (laughed) I always thought of just little babies nursing, but never older children. I thought I'll breastfeed for a year, but I'm not really sure I'm going to do anything after that.

When asked to detail how they came to breastfeed beyond their child's first year birthday, most of these mothers stated that during their pregnancy they had planned to breastfeed but were thinking of weaning completely from the breast between six months and a year. By the time the six-month period had ended, most knew other mothers who were breastfeeding toddlers. For some mothers, this experience occurred at a La Leche League meeting. Other mothers knew a close friend or relative who was engaged in extended breastfeeding. Conversations about the topic often ensued. As they became more familiar with the practice and their children approached a year of age and showed no interest in weaning, the mothers continued breastfeeding. Often their timetable for weaning was repeatedly extended. This practice evolved as their child grew and they became familiar with extended breastfeeding.

Reasons for continuing breastfeeding. The Hispanic mothers' primary motivation to continue breastfeeding beyond a year of age was generally based on nutritional and health reasons.

In contrast, the non-Hispanic mothers repeatedly identified providing nurturance or comfort to the child. Near the end of the child's first year, the non-Hispanic mothers stated that breastfeeding became primarily a means of giving comfort to the child during periods of stress and fatigue, and maintaining intimacy between the mother and a very active toddler.

The non-Hispanic mothers cited other advantages. Although many of the mothers were advised to give formula if they weaned their child from the breast prior to a year of age, they found that the nutritional and health advantages of breastfeeding, in addition to its convenience, outweighed having to deal with formula and bottles for the first year. As these non-Hispanic mothers became familiar with advantages of continuing to breastfeed, and as their children seemed to "enjoy it," they saw no reason to wean.

By the end of the child's first year, the non-Hispanic mothers described their difficulty refusing the breast to children who were old enough developmentally to make clear by words or actions what they wanted. Many of the mothers who attempted weaning from the breast at this age described the process as extremely challenging. The mothers saw no reason to wean their child from something they both enjoyed.

Both the Hispanic and non-Hispanic mothers described extended breastfeeding as a "natural" choice for the mother and the child and one promoting mother-child attachment. They expressed experiencing a deeper level of intimacy through physical contact with their child while breastfeeding. This made them feel more responsive to other needs of their child. They described breastfeeding as reinforcing closeness between them and their child.

Although both the Hispanic and non-Hispanic mothers described extended breastfeeding as "natural," the word appeared to have different meanings to the two groups. For example, several Hispanic mothers based their choice to continue breastfeeding upon a natural common custom. One mother, who had been nursed as a young child, stated:

In my country some childs [sic] are breastfed until they are two-years-old. It is very common. It's just something that happens. I just remember that it's very natural there. You just lift up your blouse anywhere you are, and you feed the baby there.

The non-Hispanic mothers used "natural" to describe as the choice to continue breastfeeding, not only from their perspective but also from the child's. One mother stated, "It's the natural choice. It's the choice the child wants." The term was also prevalent in their discussion of child-led weaning, a process by which the child provides cues for feedings and the time of weaning. In contrast, the term "artificial" emerged in the mothers' discussions of formula and the use of bottles. For the non-Hispanic group, the discussion of "natural" pervaded other aspects of mothering, such as home birthing, home schooling, eating natural foods, toilet training, carrying or wearing the baby, using homeopathic medicines, and natural family planning.

The non-Hispanic mothers repeatedly described closeness to their child as being "in tune with" or keyed into what their child needed. This flexible style of mothering pervaded other aspects of parenting, such as allowing their child to move at their own pace, whether it be the introduction of solid foods or toilet training.

Three of the mothers (2 Hispanic and 1 non-Hispanic) were practicing extended breastfeeding because of their child's intolerance to formula and milk products or refusal to accept other drink or solids when weaning from the breast was attempted.

Concealment of the practice. When asked about any disadvantages of extended breastfeeding, both Hispanic and non-Hispanic mothers frequently addressed their perception of a social stigma against the practice. Many elaborated on specific circumstances in which they encountered a negative reaction to their continued breastfeeding. A non-Hispanic mother discussed an incident in which she was reprimanded for breast-feeding her 18-month-old male toddler in public:

> But for me, the feelings of embarrassment I had to overcome were significant. The concerns I had about being seen nursing even in my own back yard. . . Just the idea of being cited as a nursing pair with him past the baby age was a great concern.

In response to these negative sanctions, many of the non-Hispanic mothers adopted some form of "closet nursing," breastfeeding with some degree of secrecy. They also encouraged their child to use a code word such as "na na" for breast-feeding. The mothers found this helpful in public situations, where others were unaware of their child's request to nurse.

When the Hispanic mothers were questioned about their perception of the differences in continuing to breastfeed between their country of origin and the United States, all of the women recognized that they were going "against the norm" of the United States. One mother stated,

The current emphasis of clinical research on lactation as a source of nutrients rather than as a nurturing process may be a contributing factor towards the lack of research interest in the area of extended breastfeeding.

"When I came here I realized that this country was very diverse with many people of different backgrounds, so I don't expect people to agree with what I do or what I believe." Many stated they had been encouraged to wean by health professionals, friends, and even family members, who lived outside their primary household. However, neither "closet nursing" nor the use of a code word were practices identified by the Hispanic mothers. When questioned about the prevalence of these practices among Hispanics, several mothers expressed surprise and initial difficulty understanding why a mother would use such practices.

Sources of support. The Hispanic mothers most often recognized breastfeeding peer counselors as their major source of support for extended breastfeeding. In contrast, the non-Hispanic mothers identified two primary sources of support for extended breastfeeding: their spouses, who provided emotional support, and La Leche League members, who contributed informational support (see Table 4). Neither group of mothers identified their own mothers or health professionals as primary sources of support for continued breastfeeding.

Conclusions

Nourishment vs. Nurturance. In discussing the primary purpose of long-term breastfeeding, the Hispanic mothers focused primarily on nutritional and health reasons (nourishment). They viewed continued breastfeeding as closely linked to their child's biological growth and development and their health status. The non-

Table 4. Primary Sources of Support for Extended Breastfeeding

Source of Support	Hispanic (n = 10)	Non-Hispanic (n = 30)
Spouse	20%	47%
Peer counselor	40%	0%
La Leche League member	0%	30%
Female friend	0%	17%
Sister	0%	3%
Sister-in-law	0%	3%
Mother-in-law	10%	0%

Hispanic mothers believed that breast-feeding a toddler provided more than calories for growth or antibodies for continued health but was an important way of meeting the emotional needs of the child. They viewed extended breastfeeding as "nurturance," an important contribution to their child's emotional development.

The meaning of breastfeeding as nourishment and nurturance is comparable to Van Esterik's (1985) conceptual differentiation between breastfeeding as "product" or "process." All the women in this study identified breast-milk as a nutritional pro-duct providing nourishment. They discussed its attributes, such as optimal nutrition and anti-infective properties, which contributed toward their child's healthfulness. Bottle-fed infants were perceived as prone to more episodes of illness than breastfed infants.

In addition to describing breastmilk as a product, many of the non-Hispanic mothers emphasized the nurturing process of breast-feeding. They viewed prolonged breastfeeding as creating a special bonding relationship between mother and child. Substituting infant formula in a bottle for the complex process of breastfeeding was seen as more than a decision about the relative cost or nutritional value of the two products or the practical convenience of the two processes. When breastmilk held more than nutritional importance and was thought of as a process that provided contact and comfort, bottle-feeding was resisted.

Natural Mothering. Discussions of "natural mothering" prevalent in the non-Hispanic group of mothers are consistent with La Leche League's view of an overall style of mothering (Weiner, 1994). La Leche League has long favored extended breastfeeding as a means of enhancing the emotional and physical health of the child by permitting the child, rather than a health care provider, to determine the duration of breastfeeding and the timing of weaning from the breast. The idea that a child should set the schedule for feedings and the time of weaning continues to distinguish the League from many health care providers who promote a breastfeeding regimen directed by external standards based on time. How much of the mothers' reported trend toward natural mothering was promoted through their contact with La Leche League is unclear, since this contact varied.

An attachment style of parenting. A prevalent comment among the non-Hispanic mothers related to the closeness between the mother and child that was enhanced by extended breastfeeding. Avery (1977) suggests that by the time a breastfeeding child has reached a year of age, the mother has become thoroughly comfortable responding to the child's cues. She describes this notion of responding to the child's cues as "being attuned" to the child.

In a study of 12 women who had breastfed for over a year, Wrigley and Hutchinson (1990) identified "tuning-in" as part of the phase of "synchronization" in which a mother allows her child "to set the pace of his or her physical, emotional and social developments, while the mother uses her unique knowledge of that particular child to enhance that development" (p. 37). The mother becomes aware of the child's physical and emotional needs and "tunes-in" to the child's developmental pace. Following semi-structured in-depth interviews with their subjects, these researchers reported that the mothers made a cognitive decision not only to be with the child at all times but also to remain aware of the child and his/her movements and activities. They describe this need for close proximity as "presencing" or "the mother being near the child at all times."

Limitations

This study is limited by the sample's small size and lack of random selection. The sample may not be reflective of long-term breastfeeders because of the select nature of the population studied and their differences in employment, education, and income. The range of years of residency in the United States for the Hispanic subjects varied greatly. Furthermore, several of the non-Hispanic subjects were recruited through contacts with Leche League. It is possible that the women in contact with La Leche League may have had opinions that reflect League philosophy rather than that of the general population of long-term breastfeeders.

Although breastfeeding up to a year of age may occur frequently in Hispanic countries, it is not as common among different Hispanic subgroups in the United States (Rassin, et al., 1994). Further studies are needed to determine the differences between other populations of Hispanic and non-Hispanic mothers in respect to the long-term outcomes associated with extended breastfeeding. It would also be valuable to gain a more complete understanding about the pros and cons of the nurturance, comforting, and bonding that the non-Hispanic mothers emphasize.

These data are based on the mothers' self-reports. While the maternal perspective offers insight into the mothers' reasons for and perceptions of the breastfeeding experience, it is also possible that the mothers' evaluation of extended breastfeeding would not be supported by more controlled, independent observations.

Implications for Clinical Practice and Future Research

It is important for the lactation consultant to identify and assess a mother's primary conceptualization of extended breastfeeding, whether it be as a "product" that provides optimal nutrition and healthy antibodies or as a "process" that allows the mother to nurture the child and maintain a close intimate bond. Sensitivity to ethnicity and its relationship to mothers' motivations for continuing to breastfeed guides the counselor in giving informational or emotional support to the mother. The woman with a product orientation would most likely require a different approach when encouraged to continue breastfeeding than someone with a process orientation. Women who have primarily a "product" orientation may also value information on the nurturing benefits of extended breastfeeding as described by other mothers. And, women who especially value the "process" benefits may benefit from information regarding the nutritional and anti-infective properties of prolonged breastfeeding. Understanding the mother's orientation may help to direct the lactation consultant toward the most appropriate concerns for her client.

Educational programs for breastfeeding counselors and other health professionals needs to include information on the feasibility and benefits of breastfeeding beyond the first year. Many mothers have concerns about the short-

Educational programs for health professionals need to include information relating to the feasibility and benefits of nursing beyond the first year and its relationship to maternal concerns regarding the child's growth and development.

and long-term effects of continued breastfeeding on their child's growth and development. Other women who lack family or friends experienced with and supportive of continued breastfeeding may need counseling on the practical issues of extended breastfeeding such as how to cope with societal negative reactions, getting adequate sleep, or determining the optimal time and means of encouraging weaning by an older child.

An increasing number of women are not satisfied to live the dual existence of a "closet nurser." They refuse to conceal their behavior and express a moral and political responsibility toward other breastfeeding mothers and society to make their behavior and motivations known. More research is needed that examines ongoing events, such as the mother's evolving attitudes and beliefs towards breastfeeding a growing child at various developmental stages.

References

American Academy of Pediatrics, Work Group on Breastfeeding (1997). Breastfeeding and the use of human milk. *Pediatrics* 100 (6), 1035-7.

Avery JL (1977). Closet nursing: A symptom of intolerance and a forerunner of social change? *Keeping Abreast Journal* 2 (4), 212-7.

Bottorff JL (1990). Persistence in breastfeeding: A phenomenological investigation. *Journal of Advanced Nursing* 15, 201-9.

Buckley KM (1992). Beliefs and practices related to extended breastfeeding among La Leche League mothers: A descriptive survey. *Journal of Perinatal Education* 1, 45-53.

Dewey KG, Finley DA, Lönnerdal B (1984). Breast milk volume and composition during late lactation (7-20 months). *Journal of Pediatric Gastroenterology and Nutrition* 3 (5), 713-20.

Kendall-Tackett KA, Sugarman M (1995). The social consequences of long-term breastfeeding. *Journal of Human Lactation* 11 (3), 179-83.

Lawrence, RA (1994). *Breastfeeding: A guide for the medical profession.* St. Louis, MO: Mosby.

Miles MB, Huberman M. (1994). *Qualitative data analysis: An expanded sourcebook.* (2nd ed.) Newbury Park, CA: Sage.

Nieswiadomy RM (1998). *Foundations of Nursing Research,* Stamford, CT: Appleton & Lange, p. 127.

Rassin DK, Markides KS, Baranowski T, Richardson CJ, Mikrut WD, Bee DE. (1994). Acculturation and the initiation of breastfeeding. *Journal of Clinical Epidemiology* 47 (7), 739-46.

UNICEF/WHO (1990). *Innocenti Declaration: On the Protection, Promotion and Support of Breastfeeding.* New York: UNICEF.

US Bureau of Census (1995). *Statistical Abstract of the United States: 1995.* (115th ed.) Washington, D.C.

US Dept of Health and Human Services (1990). *Healthy People 2000; National Health Promotion and Disease Prevention Objectives.* Washington, D.C.: USGPO.

Van Esterik P (1985). Commentary: An anthropological perspective on infant feeding in Oceania: In

LB Marshall, *Infant Care and Feeding in the South Pacific,* (pp. 339-340). New York: Gordon and Breach.

Weiner LY (1994). Reconstructing motherhood: The La Leche League in postwar America. *The Journal of American History* 80, 1357-81.

Wilson-Clay B (1990). Extended breastfeeding as a legal issue: An annotated bibliography. *Journal of Human Lactation* 6 (2), 68-71.

Wrigley EA, Hutchinson SA (1990). Long-term breastfeeding: The secret bond. *Journal of Nurse-Midwifery* 35 (1), 35-41.

Signs and Superscripts

NB: *This column examines issues pertaining to research methods (how investigators collect or obtain data) and statistics (how those data are analyzed). These research elements have implications for the reported results and how these results are useful to clinicians working with breastfeeding mothers and babies. We look forward to receiving suggestions for future topics for this column from readers.*

—The Editors.

"First, Do No Harm":
Evaluating Research for Clinical Practice

Patricia J. Martens, PhD, IBCLC

Pat Martens is a researcher with the Manitoba Centre for Health Policy and Evaluation, and Assistant Professor in the Department of Community Health Sciences, Faculty of Medicine, University of Manitoba, Winnipeg, Manitoba, Canada. Her areas of interest as a researcher and a certified lactation consultant include: breastfeeding decisions of First Nations women; evaluation of community breastfeeding promotion programs; and biostatistics/research design issues. Contact the author at Manitoba Centre for Health Policy and Evaluation, Department of Community Health Sciences, University of Manitoba, R2008 – 351 Tache Avenue, Winnipeg, MB R2H 2A6 Canada.

Currents Issues in Clinical Lactation 2002, 37–47: bias, breastfeeding research, critical evaluation of research design, external validity, internal validity, validity.

Abstract

"First, do no harm" is the basis for health care provider decisions worldwide. It is essential to be a critical reader of the medical literature before attempting to apply evidence-based research findings to clinical practice. Possible research biases include: threats to internal validity (*little arrow* bias, which refers to issues of the arrow of causality); threats to external validity (*big picture* bias, which refers to generalizeability of findings); the *whodunit* bias, which refers to issues of sponsorship; face/content validity (*what-do-you-mean* bias, which refers to the definitions used and the suitability of survey content to the population being surveyed) and issues of statistical analysis decisions. Finally, rather than basing evidence on the "First, do no harm" mandate, clinicians may at times be guided by the urge to "first, do" something, despite the lack of sufficient or appropriate evidence to support the intervention. This personal bias is addressed in the *first do* bias, which refers to the suspension of critical analysis skills when faced with a possible proactive treatment option.

Introduction

"First, do no harm" is the basis for health care provider decisions worldwide. Thus, it is essential to be a critical reader of the research when you want to give your clients the most appropriate information. You want to base your practice on "evidence," but you also want to avoid doing harm by first evaluating the validity of that evidence. Evaluating research can be tedious. Before avoiding this first step to providing evidence-based care, consider the downside of *not* evaluating it: you might do harm.

How can you critique research findings? How do you know if it suits your clinical practice needs? First, recognize that there is no perfect research design. Each design has its own

"First, do no harm" is the basis for health care provider decisions worldwide.

set of biases; thus, all research must be critiqued before you apply the recommendations deriving from the results to your clinical practice. This article identifies five biases to consider when evaluating research findings: the *little arrow* bias, the *big picture* bias, the *whodunit* bias, the *what-do-you-mean* bias, and the *first do* bias. Some designs (for example, nonrandomized experiments) have more problems with internal validity, or the "little arrow" bias. Some designs considered to be the gold standard in the medical research world (for example, randomized trials) often present more problems with external validity or the "big picture" bias. Then there are the less-talked-about biases, those relating to sponsored research and statistical testing ("whodunit" bias), biases relating to the research definitions used ("what-do-you-mean" bias), and our own personal biases ("First, do" bias).

To help people think about the biases in each

We need to become the lactation consultants' equivalent of Sherlock Holmes and search the research article for clues as to competing biases and alternative explanations.

type of research design, Campbell and Stanley (1966) listed a wide variety of research designs and the types of biases to which each design may be subject. Other methodology textbooks and articles provide additional discussion of these research designs and their biases (Cook and Campbell, 1979; Carmines and Zeller, 1979; Spector, 1981; Creswell, 1994; Girden, 1996; Streiner and Norman, 1996; Leedy, 1997, Greenhalgh, 1997).

Types of Research Design Bias

The *little arrow* bias, commonly referred to as "threats to internal validity," refers to the problem of whether the intervention or treatment (X) really causes the observed outcome (Y). In terms of mathematical symbols, the little arrow refers to causality, in the shorthand form of does $X \rightarrow Y$. To answer this question, we need to become the lactation consultants' equivalent of Sherlock Holmes and search the research article for clues as to competing biases and alternative explanations. This "little arrow" bias is more likely to be a problem of non-randomized trials, like those that rely on a convenient comparison group (quasi-experiments) or those that have no control/comparison group.

Here is an example: two hospitals were involved in quasi-experimental research designed to determine if cabbage leaves (the "X" variable) helped reduce engorgement (the "Y" variable). In one hospital, women were given standard information about engorgement— feed frequently and use cold packs between

The whodunit bias *questions the hidden agendas in research, or the way in which the numbers were analyzed. Although most of us assume that researchers are an unbiased group of people, the sad reality is that we are all affected by our cultural desire for reciprocity.*

feeds and warm compresses with gentle massage just before feeds. In the other hospital, women were told to apply cabbage leaves to reduce their breast engorgement. The cabbage leaves seemed to be effective in reducing the engorgement. But there may be other (competing) reasons why women in the second hospital reported reduced engorgement. Perhaps staff in the hospital where cabbage leaf treatment was used also taught a technique that may relieve engorgement, such as breast massage, which was not taught at the control hospital. If so, a competing explanation may have been responsible for an outcome of reduced engorgement. Perhaps those people who participated in the research at the intervention site volunteered. Volunteers are apt to be more highly motivated women, who may also be more likely to breastfeed more frequently. Thus their more frequent breastfeeding may be the reason for reduced engorgement, not the application of cabbage leaves. Perhaps the extra attention of the staff during the research trial was enough to encourage the women to believe that there was less pain or less swelling when breastfeeding occurred. Perhaps the persons who measured degree of maternal breast engorgement were rating differently at each site or were slightly biased by expecting cabbage leaves to be more effective than other methods of reducing engorgement. On the other hand, perhaps most of these competing explanations can be ruled out, and you are convinced by the research that X really DID produce Y!

Table 1 (see pp. 41–43) summarizes threats to possible internal validity, so-called *little arrow* biases, including history, maturation, testing, instrumentation, statistical regression, selection bias, loss to follow-up differences, and temporality of X and Y (direction of the arrow). All of these elements can be summed up in one question: is there any *other* reason for the results? Put another way, do you have faith in the conclusion that X really did produce Y? Table 2 (see pp. 44–45) offers a checklist of the biases discussed and examples illustrating each bias.

"Threats to external validity" represent the *big picture* bias. In this case the question is, would the same outcome effect (Y) be seen when an intervention (X) is applied to the real world of everyday clients in an everyday clinical setting? Despite being considered the gold standard in the medical research world, the randomized trial often experiences problems with the *big picture* bias. This bias relates to the degree of "naturalness" of the circumstances. Do the people eligible for enrollment in the study truly represent most people who would seek help in your clinic? Is the experiment so rigid or so interventive that

if people were to try the treatment in a natural setting, different results might be seen? Is the treatment too difficult or too undesirable to be translated into real-world settings? Did the study subjects receive supervision, information, and follow-up far beyond what clients in the real world would normally receive? All these *big picture* biases may result in very different results when the trial treatment is applied in a natural clinical setting.

The *whodunit bias* questions the hidden agendas in research, or the way in which the numbers were analyzed. Although most of us assume that researchers are an unbiased group of people, the sad reality is that we are all affected by our cultural desire for reciprocity. That is, if someone does something good for me, I should then do something good for that person. If someone gives me money to conduct my research study, I may want to reciprocate in some way. I might feel uncomfortable if the outcome of my research work were to find that this company's product is either doing nothing or doing harm. If research involves sponsorship, it is essential that the reader carefully critique the research reported. What definitions were used? In what way might the results be interpreted differently?

Moreover, the statistical decisions made in the analysis phase of the research work also need to be evaluated. Were the most appropriate statistical tests selected? Were the sample sizes adequate to ensure a statistically significant finding? Be especially cautious when results show "no statistically significant difference," since this finding could be due to a poor

Table 1. Checklist for "Little Arrow" Sources of Bias (Threats to Internal Validity)

Biases to consider	What this means	Example
The little arrow bias: does X→Y	**Internal validity**	
• History	Did something other than X occur between the first and second measurement	In a study of prenatal class effectiveness in teaching the benefits of breastfeeding, the control group was the first class in the year, and the intervention group was the second class. However, a national TV ad campaign was aired to promote breastfeeding during the second class time period.
• Maturation	Did something change just as a function of time (healing over time, getting older)?	Women who were experiencing cracked nipples were issued a substance to apply to their nipples. They reported whether their nipples healed within a week. But this healing could also have occurred as a result of "tincture of time."
• Testing	Did the fact that people were measured or tested change their results on the second measure or test?	Because people were asked an attitude question on a pretest, they may be more likely to have different attitude scores on a posttest.
• Instrumentation	Did the measuring instrument change, or the measurer change in the way things were measured, over time?	The person evaluating the degree of engorgement on day 3 became more reliable at the task as the trial proceeded. The people enrolled in the trial received treatment A in the first 3 months, and treatment B in the second 3 months. Thus, bias occurs by the way in which engorgement was measured, rather than by the treatment studied.
• Statistical regression	Were groups initially selected on the basis of extreme scores— high or low (these high/low groups tend to become closer to the medium score over time)?	A group at high risk of weaning (scoring high on a pretest during pregnancy) were compared to those scoring medium, to see the effect of a teaching program. The high-risk group would probably score lower on a posttest. It would be better to select both the control and the intervention from the same high-risk group.
• Selection bias	Were the two groups for comparison selected differently?	

Table 1. Checklist for "Little Arrow" Sources of Bias (Threats to Internal Validity) (Continued)

Biases to consider	What this means	Example
• Loss to follow-up differences and response rate differences	Did the two groups differ as to who was to be enrolled, contacted for the follow-up, or who quit during the research?	In a follow-up study of prenatal breast-feeding classes, women were telephoned at six months postpartum to measure the duration of breastfeeding. People in the "control" group were difficult to find, and only 30% responded. In the intervention group, 80% were interviewed. The effect of the breast-feeding class may be understated, owing to an overestimate of breastfeeding duration in the control group because mobility occurred less frequently in one group.
• Direction of the arrow	In studies at one point in time, where people are recalling events, did X cause Y or did Y cause X (timing of events)?	In a cross-sectional study, you notice a correlation between bottle-feeding and confused suck at the breast. But which came first? Did the introduction of bottle-feeding produce a poor suck pattern, or did a poor suck pattern lead to problems at the breast and subsequent introduction of bottle-feeding?
• Diffusion of the information	Did the information diffuse between groups; i.e., did groups communicate with one another or did one group learn the information from the other about what worked best?	Women were randomized to receive instructions to feed on only one breast per feed versus two breasts per feed in the postpartum ward. But women in adjoining beds may compare notes and talk with one another.
• Compensatory equalization	If the good or service is desirable, there may emerge administrative reluctance to tolerate the inequality of group assignment, and "help out" the control group.	Some women received a new treatment to relieve breast engorgement, but the nursing staff also suggested the same treatment to those in the control group who needed help.
• Rivalry	The control group, as a natural underdog, may be motivated to change the expected difference through social competition.	One hospital ward was given education on BFHI; another ward was not. The other ward became aware of this, and began a competition to improve their own practices in accordance with BFHI standards
• Resentful demoralization	If an experiment is obvious and one group gets no treatment or inferior treatment, the second group may perform even poorer than expected owing to demoralization.	Staff on one ward is given extra education, and staff on the other is not. Because of resentment, the staff on the control ward performs even worse than expected.

Table 1. Checklist for "Little Arrow" Sources of Bias (Threats to Internal Validity) (Continued)

Biases to consider	What this means	Example
• Placebo effect	Despite an inactive treatment, the belief in something being done will result in changes in the group.	A nurse teaches a woman how to relieve breast engorgement using a new technique. Even if the technique is totally ineffective, the woman's belief in "doing something" may result in observed or perceived differences
• Non-blinding	Are the clients and the assessors unaware of the group assignment?	In a study of the degree of healing of cracked nipples, the assessor was aware of each client's assignment to receive treatment or not.

Table 2. Checklist of Biases, Their Meaning, and Illustrative Examples

Biases to consider	What this means	Example
The big picture	**External validity**	
• Reactivity to testing	The fact that clients are being tested or measured may make this different from a routine non-tested situation	A pretest and posttest is given to prenatal class members; a difference is noted in breastfeeding attitude scores. But this difference may occur because the class members were aware that testing was being done. This finding may not be replicated in non-tested prenatal class clients.
• Multiple treatments	If more than one treatment is being given, the results may be affected by non-erasable effects. Thus, the results cannot be generalized when only one of the treatments is provided.	In a prenatal instruction experiment, the intervention consisted of an extra breast-feeding class and assignment of a breastfeeding mentor to each class member. A public health unit wanted to begin a mentorship program, but these study results will only generalize to a situation where both interventions (the class and the mentor) are provided.
• Who was enrolled in the study?	Do the clients in this research reflect the clients in your practice? How were the subjects recruited? Were they volunteers? Who was included or excluded by the criteria in the study?	Clients from a low-income group of a certain ethnicity who gave birth to full-term infants are asked to volunteer for an experiment. The study findings may not be generalizable to high-income women, those of different ethnic groups, women giving birth to preterm infants, or to people who would not volunteer to participate.

Table 2. Checklist of Biases, Their Meaning, and Illustrative Examples (Continued)

Biases to consider	What this means	Example
The big picture	**External validity**	
• Is this the "real world"?	Were the people in this experiment getting treatment they would normally receive, or "extra-special" treatment, observation, follow-up, and equipment?	People enrolled in a trial to observe the effects of a new drug on mastitis were given detailed, lengthy explanations for treating mastitis, contact information for 24-hour a day help if needed, and assistance with child-care during the trial. This new drug may seem to be more beneficial than if only the drug is provided.
Whodunit bias		
• Sponsorship bias	Is there a corporate interest in seeing certain results, and has the research been sponsored by this corporate interest?	A company that markets infant formula sponsors research on the health differences of breastfed and formula-fed babies, but the sample size may be too small to detect a statistically significant difference.
• Statistician bias	Are the sample sizes big enough to detect a clinically significant difference if it exists? Are the statistical tests correctly chosen and correctly used?	A trial to see if there is a difference in breastfeeding duration between groups receiving peer counseling versus regular public health contacts has a limited sample size. Even though the counselled group breastfeeds longer, the effect is not statistically significant and the conclusion is "no difference."
What-do-you-mean bias	(Face validity, construct validity, content validity)	
• Consider the definitions used	Do the definitions make sense—for example, how is "breastfeeding" defined?	In a study comparing the health differences of breastfed and non-breastfed infants, "breastfed" means breastfed for at least 1 month; "non-breastfed" includes babies who were initially breastfed for up to 1 month, thus diluting the difference between the groups
• Consider the outcomes measured	What is the outcome measure and is this an appropriate measure of success?	In a study to detect the effect of exercise on breastfeeding experiences, the outcome measure was lactic acid concentration levels in breastmilk. Is the investigator more interested in an outcome measure of breast refusal by the infant?

Table 2. Checklist of Biases, Their Meaning, and Illustrative Examples (Continued)

Biases to consider	What this means	Example
The big picture	External validity	
First DO bias		
• Evaluate your own bias	When you see a new treatment, do you jump on the bandwagon and suspend your critiquing skills in order to *do* something for your clients?	You see a new treatment for helping with cracked nipples, based on one anecdotal case study. You want to try it with your clients in order to offer something to them.
• Self-validation bias	Do you only look for research articles that verify your own pre-conceived notions?	You are convinced that a certain treatment works for increasing milk supply. You do a literature search and select those articles that show a positive effect, and you ignore those articles whose findings do not support your view.
• Publication bias	Publishers of research journals also tend to bias what is published—it is more interesting to publish positive results than results that show no difference.	When doing a review of the literature, be aware that published studies finding "no difference" may be under-represented. Search for other sources of information on intervention results, such as conference proceedings.

research design with too few participants enrolled in the study (Martens, 1995).

"Face validity," "construct validity," and "content validity" is the *what-do-you-mean* bias. Do the research definitions make sense? Use your experience and your clinical knowledge to approach this question and others that follow. Are the survey questions meaningful to the people of whom they are asked, or has this survey been validated using one population and then applied to a markedly different population? For example, were the survey questions tested using well-educated Caucasian women and then used in a low-income, lower education group whose members may not understand the questions in the same way? Do the survey questions really measure what they are intended to measure? For example, does a survey designed to measure a person's "breastfeeding confidence" make sense to you? Does the outcome measure something that makes sense in terms of the research reported and in terms of your clients?

Biases *We* Bring to the Research Party

You may, at this point, be questioning whether any researcher can be trusted to provide findings (that all-important evidence) on which to base your clinical practice. We, however, may be are our own worst enemy! The bias to which we may *all* be guilty is the *"First, Do"* bias—in spite of the fact that it is not found in any official list of research biases. When you read a journal article describing some new invention or treatment to alleviate a certain breastfeeding problem, you may *want* to believe it. After all, lactation consultants want to be able to *do* something for their clients. Thus, we may suspend all critical analysis and apply the treatment without reminding ourselves of the rest of the phrase . . . "First, *do no harm.*" Before falling into this trap, force yourself to sit down, read the entire article, and don the Sherlock Holmes hat. Try to find as many flaws as you can—the *little arrow*, the *big picture*, the *who-dunit*, the *what-do-you-mean* biases—and applaud yourself for being a superlative detective. After you have been ruthlessly critical of the research study, put all the pieces back together again and make an informed decision.

Do you accept that the intervention X really "caused" the outcome Y? Are the findings applicable to the people with whom you work? Will this new treatment be more effective than your current practice, knowing all the flaws of the study that you have identified? Is there potential for harm if you change your practice on the basis of the evidence you have just reviewed? Is more research needed to convince you of the benefits of the practices that the investigators recommend? And, if so, how might you conduct some of that research or inspire others to do so?

Tables 1 and 2 contain checklists of biases and points to consider to help you in your role

The bias to which we may all be guilty is the First, Do *bias—in spite of the fact that it is not found in any official list of research biases. When you read a journal article describing some new invention or treatment to alleviate a certain breastfeeding problem, you may* want *to believe it. After all, lactation consultants want to be able to do* something for their clients.

as the Sherlock Holmes of breastfeeding research. You must be a detective if you are to *appropriately* apply evidence-based care in your clinical practice. Why? Because you need to live by the mandate of "First, do no harm," even as you realize your potential to extend the know-ledge boundaries of the lactation consultant profession.

References

Campbell DT, Stanley JC (1966). *Experimental and quasi-experimental designs for research.* Dallas: Houghton Mifflin.

Carmines EG, Zeller RA (1979). *Reliability and Validity Assessment.* Sage University Paper Series on Quantitative Applications in the Social Sciences, Series No. 07-017. Newbury Park, CA: Sage, pp.17-27.

Cook TD, Campbell DT (1979). *Quasi-Experimentation: Design & Analysis Issues for Field Settings.* Boston: Houghton Mifflin, pp. 37-146.

Creswell JW (1994). *Research Design: Qualitative & Quantitative Approaches.* Thousand Oaks, CA: Sage, pp. 116-42.

Girden ER (1996). *Evaluating Research Articles from Start to Finish.* Thousand Oaks, CA: Sage, pp.1-21.

Greenhalgh T (1997). How to read a paper: Assessing the methodological quality of published papers. *British Medical Journal* 315 (2 August): 305-308.

Leedy PD (1997). *Practical Research: Planning and Design,* Columbus, OH: Prentice-Hall, pp.229-42.

Martens PJ (1995). A mini-lesson in statistics: what causes treatment groups to be deemed 'not statistically different'? *Journal of Human Lactation* 11(2):117-121.

Spector PE (1981). *Research Designs.* Sage University Paper Series on Quantitative Applications in the Social Sciences, Series No. 07-023. Newbury Park, CA: Sage, pp.14-78.

Streiner DL, Norman GR (1996). *PDQ Epidemiology,* 2nd ed. Toronto: Mosby, pp. 29-78.

The Business of Clinical Practice

NB: *This column highlights one or more settings where lactation scientists and clinicians work, to suggest how lactation consulting can be integrated into similar settings. This issue describes a lactation clinic housed in a referral children's hospital. Suggestions for other practice settings to highlight in future issues of CICL should be sent to the Editorial Office.*

Development of a Regional Tertiary Lactation Service in a Children's Hospital

Anne Mercer, RN, MSN, IBCLC

Anne Mercer is a lactation consultant and clinical coordinator for Childen's Mercy Hospitals and Clinics, Kansas City, Missouri. Contact the author at Lactation Program, Children's Mercy Hospitals and Clinics, 2401 Gillham Road, Kansas City, MO 64108 USA.

Currents Issues in Clinical Lactation 2002, 49–53; children's hospital, hospitalized infants, NICU, preterm infants, referral practice.

Small Beginnings

Children's Mercy Hospital now has a lactation program. At its outset, our aim was to enhance the quality and amount of support for health professionals and the families whose babies were in the neonatal intensive care unit (NICU).

In 1991, Children's Mercy was involved with the Wellstart International Program. We sent a neonatologist, neonatal nutritionist, and neo-

> *Our aim was to enhance the quality and amount of support for health professionals and the families whose babies were in the Neonatal Intensive Care Unit (NICU).*

natal nurse practitioner to the "Train the Trainer" program in San Diego. Prior to receiving approval to provide such a service, two NICU staff nurses and a neonatal nurse prac-titioner (NNP) collected information from families whose babies had been cared for in our NICU. Breastfeeding initiation at that time hovered around 40%. Other information included how many mother/baby dyads were being helped per shift, how much time staff were spending with these patients per shift, what problems were being addressed, what supplies were needed to continue this care, and discharge information, which included infant diagnoses and whether interventions offered were influencing the babies' length of stay. Data from the parents also were gathered concerning their response to the lactation assistance received, whether they felt that rooming-in prior to the baby's discharge would have been helpful and information pertaining to the use of electric or manual breast pumps. Wellstart personnel supported our proposal for a lactation program. In 1993, our program began with funding for one fulltime and one part-time lactation consultant position.

Initial Services

We first offered consultations to the patients in the NICU. These services included breast pump rentals for mothers whose babies were not yet able to breastfeed, assisting with initiation of breastfeeding when the infants were clinically stable, and discharge follow-up in the outpatient lactation clinic, as needed. After this

program was in place, staff from the infant toddler unit, pediatric intensive care unit (PICU), and the infectious disease unit began requesting assistance with breast-feeding infants in their care. In 1993, breast pumps on trolleys were purchased and placed in these units. A breast pumping room was set up for the mothers whose babies were in the NICU. In addition, a lactation help line phone number was established for mothers in the community and former patients' mothers to use. We provided this number to personnel in referring hospitals as well.

Growth of the Service

In 1995, a parttime lactation coordinator was added to our staff to assist with outreach and staff education. At this time, we had one full-time lactation consultant (LC), one parttime LC, and one parttime lactation coordinator.

In 1997, we began offering three meals a day to all mothers who were breastfeeding their hospitalized infants. Breastfeeding mothers previously had been expected to buy their meals from the cafeteria or to have family members bring food in for them. This same year, after the NICU was moved to a new location in the hospital, the lactation team was provided with a breast pumping room equipped with dim lights, four electric breast pumps, curtains to provide privacy for each pumping station (if desired), a sink in which to wash equipment, and a small radio/CD/tape player. And, in 1998 another half-time position was added to the lactation team. Freezer space is provided for storing breastmilk for infants in the NICU and PICU. All other units within the hospital now have at least one electric breast pump for breastfeeding mothers to use. In 2000, the Emergency Room also received a breast pump for the mothers in their unit. Previously, mothers in the ER had to make do with a manual pump unless a member of the lactation team was available to bring a portable pump to these mothers.

Current Services

Our NICU has 40 beds. We usually see 20-25 patients in the NICU daily. We can also handle between 3 and 20 patients per day outside the NICU. These services are offered from 8AM to 5PM Monday through Friday and for four hours on Sunday. We are on call 24 hours a day, 7 days a week. Our guidelines govern when we come in for consults at times other than when the service is usually provided. In 1996, we opened a small retail program to provide portable breast pumps. This service was expanded to include sales of bras in 1998. Sales from this program help to offset our costs.

We see babies representing a wide variety of challenges, including preterm infants, ill fullterm infants such as those with a cleft palate/lip or cardiac conditions, post-surgical patients, and babies with congenital defects, necrotizing enterocolitis, and a variety of syndromes. We also serve mothers in the community with fullterm infants whose needs may or may not represent a high-risk situation.

We are gratified that our breastfeeding initia-

We see babies representing a wide variety of challenges, including preterm infants, ill fullterm infants such as those with a cleft palate/lip or cardiac conditions, post-surgical patients, and babies with congenital defects, necrotizing enterocolitis, and a variety of syndromes.

tion rate in the NICU has grown from 40% to 75%. I attribute our increased breastfeeding rate to the support of these mothers and babies by the lactation team, staff nurses, and physicians at all levels and in all units. Being part of the lactation program at this Children's Hospital has been exciting and challenging. I accomplish something new each day! Our work is truly worth the effort.

Requirements for Serving on the Lactation Team

All members of the lactation team must have at least a Bachelor of Science in Nursing (BSN) degree, and IBLCE certification (preferred). These requirements were established when the lactation consultant was hired in 1995. A neonatologist serves as the lactation team's medical director. This person does not have IBLCE certification. Currently, we have one fulltime consultant, two parttime consultants, and two as-needed consultants on staff. [As demands for our service have increased, staff has been added. In a perfect world, I would like to have one or two more fulltime LCs as well as milk technicians in the NICU to prepare the breastmilk for the staff to give to the babies.]

Referrals

We receive referrals from community hospitals as well as pediatricians. As our residents move into practice, they refer patients back to us. In the hospital, we contact all mothers whose babies have been admitted to the NICU to determine if they have begun providing breastmilk for their babies. The mother of any baby admitted outside the NICU also receives a courtesy call to inform her of our services, to answer any questions she might have, and to assist them as needed. Physicians can also order a lactation consult. Our services also are advertised by our hospital referral line and by word of mouth.

Persons who wish to develop a similar program need to gather statistics, have a proposal that makes clear how the program will impact the particular setting where it will exist—whether that is in a general hospital, office or private practice, or a referral hospital.

Community Service

Our program is one of five in the area. Ours is a referral hospital; none of the babies we care for are born at our institution. Therefore, we depend on staff at the referring hospitals to help the mother with initiation of pumping when their babies are not yet able to go to the breast. When a baby is transferred to our unit and breast pumping or breastfeeding has already begun, we depend on the staff at the referring hospital to initiate such activities unless the mother has been discharged. If she is discharged, we help her initiate breast pumping or breastfeeding when she arrives. When a baby is admitted to another unit in our hospital and is already breastfeeding, we assist in its continuation or breast pumping, depending on the circumstances of the mother-baby pair. We support the programs at other hospitals by offering regional outreach education to the community health care professionals.

Future Plans

Currently, the lactation team offers an annual basic lactation workshop. This year, we will offer a regional intermediate-level workshop. Over the next five years, we propose to request a position for a breastmilk technician in the NICU to preparing feedings, monitor storage and thawing of breastmilk, and preparation of the milk 24 hours a day. The technician will prepare the milk for gavage feedings or any other feedings when the mother is not available to feed her baby. We also would like to initiate breastmilk/breastfeeding studies. Over the next ten years, our goal is to continue to expand our services in the community through the out-patient clinic, within the hospital, and to participate in research studies.

Advice to Others

Persons who wish to develop a similar program need to gather statistics and have a proposal that makes clear how the program will impact the particular setting where it will exist—whether that is in a general hospital, office or private practice, or a referral hospital. Each staff member should be prepared to put in many hours until the program is established. Seek backup support and give credit for every little success. Don't put down personnel or the program when things look difficult. If staff find themselves with no support from others, program goals and the mission need to be reevaluated.

The three most important skills a person needs to start such a program are the ability and willingness to communicate with and listen to others, patience, and business skills. The greatest impediments most programs are likely to encounter are financial (the cost of running the program) and staffing. One person cannot do it all, and dependable, skilled staff is essential.

Commentary

Preterm Infants and Mothers: The Need for Long-term Breastfeeding Support

Roberta J. Hewat, PhD, RN, IBCLC

Roberta Hewat is an Assistant Professor in the School of Nursing, University of British Columbia, 2211 Wesbrook Mall, Vancouver, BC V6T 3B5 Canada.

Current Issues in Clinical Lactation, 2002, 55–57; breastfeeding support, evidence-based practice, mother, preterm infants.

Breastfeeding is a challenge to the mothers of preterm infants and their caregivers, yet research findings and information about programs to assist this population with breastfeeding based on clinical evidence is limited. Two manuscripts in this issue focus on this important topic. One is a study, well executed, on pre-mature infants' feeding patterns for 10 weeks after discharge from a Neonatal Intensive Care Unit (NICU) (Piper, 2001). The second describes a successful program, initiated in a NICU, to assist breastfeeding mothers (Mercer, 2001). Although they represent different kinds of literature, both contribute knowledge for evidence-based practice.

Investigation of infant feeding patterns for 10 weeks following an infant's discharge from a NICU is the focus of the study by Piper. Of importance is the method in which the patterns were examined. An intensity ratio was generated for determining the proportion of breastmilk feedings (from the breast or expressed breastmilk) to other liquid feedings fed to the infant. This measure is useful for comparing the intensity of breastmilk feedings and changes in the infants' feeding patterns over time. A further delineation of the ratio into categories of full, high, medium, low, and no breastmilk exposure, congruent with those of the Inter-agency Group for Action on Breastfeeding (Labbok and Krasovec, 1990), allows more precise examination of the infant feeding patterns.

Of great concern is the study finding that although all mothers had intended to breastfeed their infants before and after hospital discharge, 42% of the infants were not receiving any breastmilk at discharge, and this percentage increased to 67% by 10 weeks post discharge. Of further interest is the author's discovery that the intensity ratio for breastmilk feedings was highest at two weeks following discharge. As indicated by the author, this supports Kavenaugh et al.'s (1995) finding that two weeks after hospital discharge appears to be a "turning point" in a mother's concerns about her premature infant's breastmilk intake. The delineation of infant feeding patterns in the first 10 weeks after NICU discharge shows a significant decline of breastfeeding during this time period. This evidence identifies the need for long-term interventions and programs for assisting women with breastfeeding their pre-

term infants during as well as after their baby's discharge from a NICU.

The second manuscript describes a lactation service that was initiated in 1993 to increase the quality of breastfeeding support in a NICU for both staff and mothers of preterm infants. The dual purpose of enhancing breastfeeding support for both staff and mothers unquestionably contributes to the success of the program, which now has been extended to assist mothers of full term infants with special conditions who are hospitalized.

Further expansion of the service includes education inservices, an annual workshop, and outreach presentations at other hospitals in the geographic area. These ongoing educational programs to update knowledge undoubtedly also contribute to enhancing positive attitudes to breastfeeding among staff; such positive attitudes very likely further effect quality care and encouragement for breastfeeding mothers. The increase in breastfeeding initiation rates in the NICU from 40% to 70% since the program was started is an achievement to be celebrated.

A combination of many factors may contribute to the success of this program: the motivation, energies, and foresight of the initiators; the variety of disciplines involved from the beginning; and, continued support from administration throughout the years. All persons involved are to be congratulated for sustaining and expanding this program. However, evaluation of the program is needed to analyze more fully its strengths, benefits, and limitations, and to determine additional outcomes related to staff education and satisfaction of mothers. Documentation of the effectiveness of the program will provide stronger evidence for use in other clinical settings and may highlight elements of the program that need to be expanded or improved.

Elements of both manuscripts offer insights and contribute to the current knowledge for building strategies that assist mothers and their premature infants—a uniquely vulnerable population—with breastfeeding. We have learned several things from these articles:

a) the important aspects of a successful breastfeeding program in a NICU;

b) that breastfeeding initiation rates among women with preterm infants can be increased when a comprehensive program is implemented;

c) that infant's breastfeeding patterns are variable after discharge from a NICU;

d) that two weeks after discharge, there is a general increase in breastfeeding among this population; and,

e) that breastfeeding declines at six and 10 weeks post discharge. This latter finding is evidence of the need of long-term breastfeeding support after NICU discharge.

The importance of these articles is not only the new information that we glean from them but also our recognition of how much more we need to learn examine, and document to enable us to provide care that is based on the best evidence possible.

References

Kavanaugh K, Mead L, Meier P, Mangurten H (1995). Getting enough: mothers' concerns about breastfeeding a premature infant after discharge. *Journal of Obstetric, Gynecologic, and Neonatal Nursing* 24(1), 23-32.

Labbok MH, Krasovec K (1990). Towards consistency in breastfeeding definitions. *Studies in Family Planning* 21(4), 226-30.

Mercer A (2002) Development of a lactation service at a tertiary regional children's hospital. In KG Auerbach, *Current Issues in Clinical Lactation 2002*. Sudbury, MA: Jones and Bartlett Publishers, pp. 35-38.

Piper S (2002) Feeding patterns of preterm infants post NICU discharge. In KG Auerbach, *Current Issues in Clinical Lactation 2002*. Sudbury MA: Jones and Bartlett Publishers, pp. 9-16.

Professional Development

A Reporting Tool to Facilitate Community-based Follow-up for At-risk Breastfeeding Dyads At Hospital Discharge

Barbara Wilson-Clay, BSEd, IBCLC and
Bernadette M. Maloney, RNC, MSN, IBCLC

Barbara Wilson-Clay has been a LLL Leader since 1982 and a lactation consultant in private practice with Austin Lactation Associates since 1987. Wilson-Clay has participated in numerous coalitions related to lactation and maternal child health. She represented ILCA as their delegate to the IBLCE and served as a member of the Certification and Ethics committees. Contact the author at 12710 Burson, Manchaca, TX 78652 USA.

Bernadette Maloney is Coordinator of Women's Health Education at St. Davids Medical Center, Austin, Texas, where she supervises the lactation and childbirth education programs.

Current Issues in Clinical Lactation, 2002, 59–67; at-risk breastfeeding, communication tool, discharge planning, lactation, postpartum, breastfeeding support.

In the United States, vaginally delivered infants and their mothers typically are discharged from the hospital before the onset of copious lactation and, in some cases, before breastfeeding is stable. For some women, such early discharge results in breastfeeding challenges that are unassisted and sometimes even unrecognized by both mothers and health professionals.

Feeding difficulties contribute to early discontinuation of breastfeeding (Ramsey and Gisel, 1996) and to occasionally well-publicized adverse outcomes that should properly be viewed as a failure of the health care system to provide appropriate follow-up for at-risk dyads. The American Academy of Pediatrics guidelines attempt to address this issue by advising that, "When discharged <48 hours after delivery, all breastfeeding mothers and their newborns should be seen by a pediatrician or other knowledgeable health care practitioner when the newborn is 2 to 4 days of age" (AAP, 1997).

All too often, however, breastfeeding infants wait two or more weeks before their first pediatric visit. Such delays prolong the period of poor feeding, result in poor infant growth, and risk compromising maternal milk supply (Hill, Aldag, and Chatterton, 1999). This article discusses a cooperative project that developed a cost-effective, efficient method for facilitating communication between hospital-based and community-based care providers when an at-risk breastfeeding dyad is discharged. We share a new communication tool designed to prevent adverse outcomes by alerting pediatricians of the need for early follow-up care for these mothers and babies.

This article discusses a cooperative project that developed a cost-effective, efficient method for facilitating communication between hospital-based and community-based care providers when an at-risk breast-feeding dyad is discharged.

The Case That Inspired This Collaboration

This collaboration began following the birth of a baby daughter to a shy, young (26-year-old) Hispanic mother who very much wanted to breastfeed. "Delia" R.[1] had tried to nurse her first child, a son, born 5 years earlier. Much to her disappointment, she felt compelled to wean him to formula after his first pediatric visit on Day 15, when the doctor told Delia her son was a pound (456 g) below his birth weight. History repeated itself when Delia's daughter, Lola, born vaginally at term with good Apgar scores, was released on Day 3 with a weight loss greater than 8% of birth weight. Baby Lola spent most of her time at the breast but mostly slept with the nipple in her mouth. Delia was breastfeeding constantly, but Lola grew increasingly lethargic.

Delia had contact in the hospital with one of the authors (BMM) for lactation help. Owing to the hospital LC's concerns about Delia and her daughter, four follow-up phone calls were made after her discharge to inquire about breastfeeding. During these calls, Delia was asked about how things were going but did not share that she was experiencing unrelieved engorgement, nor did she consistently report that she was experiencing nipple soreness. The LC/authors speculated that the mother's shyness and cultural barriers may have contributed

[1]Pseudonyms are used for the mother and her children to protect their identity.

to Delia's reluctance to describe her problems during these follow-up calls.

As part of the hospital's routine postpartum instruction, Delia was given a log form to keep track of the baby's bowel movements and was advised to feed her baby frequently. Towards the end of the first week postpartum, the hospital LC learned that the baby was sleepy and still was passing small, dark-colored stools. Delia was instructed to report this to her pediatrician, but she did not do so.

On Day 13 postpartum, Delia and her baby saw the pediatrician for their first routine newborn check. The pediatrician was concerned about the baby's poor weight gain. He referred Delia to one of the authors (BWC), a community-based lactation consultant in private practice. On Day 17, Delia was seen in her home for a full lactation assessment. She signed a consent form permitting the LC to discuss her case with her other care providers, an ethical requirement if information about a client is to be shared. A report of the lactation assessment was faxed to the referring pediatrician and the hospital-based LCs.

Data from the LC Report

Following is an excerpt from the LC report:

". . . On Day 17, baby Lola is stalled at 6lb 10oz (the same weight noted 4 days ago at the pediatric visit). This represents a weight loss greater than 10% of birth weight. Mrs. R. experienced engorgement on Days 3-4, which was painful and unrelieved for several days, so we have no reason to suspect a primary milk pro-duction problem. The baby has normal oral anatomy, although her feeding reflexes are weak—particularly suck—probably from decreased energy. Position at breast and latch-on technique required some adjustment. Baby was able to take in only 24 ml from the right breast (by test weight on electronic scale) before becoming too fatigued to continue. Mrs. R's inverted nipples appear to be the reason the baby is having difficulty feeding. Her right nipple does draw out to some extent after manual manipulation, but the left is inverted. Some inverted nipples can be extremely difficult for newborns to manage, and the condition has been noted in the literature since the 1950s to produce "lethargic feeding" (Gunther, 1955). Mothers with inverted nipples probably should be red-flagged for at-risk breastfeeding.

Neifert (1999) supports the use of hospital grade electric breast pumps and silicone nipple shields to help evert such nipples and to provide supplemental calories to the infant until infant size/strength and nipple protractility improve. Due to her unrelieved engorgement, Mrs. R's milk supply has declined. She now has to use formula to provide supplemental calories to the baby. The baby's feeding ability is further compromised by poor energy as a result of nearly three weeks of poor intake. I am suggesting generous use of pumped milk/formula until pumping can recover the milk supply. I am hopeful there is time to do this, as there appears to be a detrimental effect of prolonged engorgement that sometimes irreversibly depresses milk production in sensitive individuals. It is instructive to note that this same scenario occurred 5 years ago when Mrs. R. attempted to breastfeed her first child.

The plan for remediation includes: Frequent feedings (at least 10 feeds/24 hrs) with one ounce of supplement (pumped milk/formula) to be delivered at the beginning of each feed to give the baby energy for improved breastfeeding. Baby is to be put to breast for 10-15 minutes on the more accessible nipple. Mother was taught to observe the difference between nutritive and non-nutritive sucking. When nutritive feeding ceases, mother is to offer a second ounce of supplement. The 24-hour milk needs of the baby are calculated to be 19.5 oz. The supplementation schedule described here will provide a guaranteed 20 oz (570 ml) per day delivered by alternative feeding methods to ensure rapid catch-up growth and recovery of birth weight. The test weight demonstrates some ability to access milk directly from the breast, which will provide extra energy and keep the baby at the breast during the intervention period. Mother is to pump to stimulate her milk supply and to draw out the nipples (especially the left). A silicone shield was supplied to assist in latching the baby to the left nipple. Mrs. R is to obtain weekly weight checks until the situation has stabilized, and the milk supply and baby's weight gain are within normal limits. Supplementation of formula will be tapered as the mother's milk supply comes up, and alternate supplemental feeding will be gradually decreased as the baby demonstrates improved intake directly from the breast."

The supplementation plan worked well.

Baby Lola recovered her birth weight within five days and began to grow at a normal rate. At first, with a rental-grade pump, Delia was able to pump only half an ounce (14.5 ml) of milk from both breasts combined. Her pumped volumes quickly improved with the extra stimulation from the pump, and she soon was able to discontinue the use of formula. As the baby's energy improved, she began to nurse efficiently on Delia's more everted nipple. Delia continued to pump the breast with the inverted nipple for several months, giving this milk to the baby by bottle. In spite of attempts to encourage Lola to nurse from the inverted nipple with the nipple shield, Lola continued to refuse that breast.

At about 4 months postpartum, Delia became discouraged when the inverted nipple became painful. She elected to wean from that breast. Delia continued nursing unilaterally on her "good" side. When contacted during the writing of this article, Delia reported that at 13 months postpartum she was still happily breastfeeding her healthy, active toddler, and was satisfied with her breastfeeding experience.

While the story of Delia's second lactation had a happy ending, it is important to remember that identical circumstances precipitated premature weaning after the birth of her son. That experience is far from unique. A study prepared by the Battelle Centers for Public Health Research and Evaluation for the U.S. Department of Agriculture suggests that many mothers face similar early breastfeeding challenges: "One-fourth of the WIC mothers who initiate breast-feeding stop by the end of the second week and one-half stop by the end of the second month. . . . During the first month after birth, only 30 percent of breastfeeding mothers have a problem-free nursing experience." (Bayday, et al, 1997) The Battelle study describes the type of problems the mothers experience, and they are problems that IBCLCs are trained to manage. Clearly, many women who require lactation help are not identified or referred in a timely manner.

One Proposed Reporting Tool

How can women like Delia be served in a more timely way, *before* their situations become desperate? The IBCLCs who were involved in Delia's case convened a meeting to consider this question. The outcome of the discussion was the creation of a rough draft of a reporting tool designed to alert the pediatrician of record (or assigned public health clinic) when a mother or infant is discharged home with risk factors identified in the literature (Neifert, 1996; Chen, et al, 1998; Alper and Manno, 1996; McBride and Danner, 1996; Chapman and Perez-Escamilla, 1999; Crowell, Hill, and Humenick, 1994; Ramsey and Gisel, 1996; Nyhan, 1952; Woolridge, 1986; Powers, 1999; Neubauer, et al, 1993; Henly, et al, 1995; Willis and Livingstone, 1995; Messner, et al, 2000; Hurst, 1996;

How can women like Delia be served in a more timely way, before *their situations become desperate?*

Hughes and Owen, 1993; Huggins, Petok, and Mireles, 2000; Neifert, Seacat, and Jobe, 1985; Livingstone and Stringer, 1999).

In the interest of efficiency, and to promote greater compliance, the reporting tool found at the end of this article was designed as a one-page faxable check list. Faxing is less expensive and time consuming than mailing, and faxing is easier than trying to reach a physician by phone. After a hospital lactation department assembles a list of fax numbers (a task that can be assigned to volunteers), the time required to complete and fax the report is minimal. The reporting form avoids assigning a diagnosis or suggesting a specific course of action. Instead, it focuses on notifying the physician of the presence of observable factors or behaviors that signal a risk for poor feeding. Completion of the report fulfills the responsibility of the hospital-based IBCLC to refer the mother and baby on for care, and transfers the responsibility of monitoring breastfeeding to the appropriate community-based care providers (IBLCE, 1999; ILCA, 1999; Lauwers and Shinskie, 2000). Space at the bottom of the form is provided for phone numbers for local breastfeeding resources.

Several draft versions of the check list were reviewed and modified after input from members of the local professional lactation consultant affiliate (The Heart of Texas Lactation Consultants Association). The document was then shared with the staff attorney of BMM's hospital, who confirmed that the wording did not imply that hospital staff had failed to address a problem.

Next, a sponsoring physician was sought to present the reporting tool at the city-wide pediatric section meeting. The monthly section meeting provides local pediatricians an opportunity to discuss practice and clinical issues and to set policy for pediatric practices at local hospitals. BMM approached the chairman of the pediatric section, who agreed to present the draft document.

Owing to questions that arose, BMM was invited to attend the next section meeting to participate in the discussion. The doctors' primary concerns related to how the LCs would use the form. It was decided that the form should be a notification only and should not be included in the infant's chart (where it was presumed that the nurses would already have recorded the feeding problems). After two reviews, the document received a consensus approval by the pediatric section (Fig. 1).

Reception of the Report Form

How is the new reporting process working? Results vary depending upon staffing and commitment to breastfeeding of the individual participating hospitals. In the LC literature, much has been written about the LC as change agent (Lauwers and Shinskie, 2000). Resistance to change is typical in institutions where it is easier to deny that a problem exists than it is to organize a plan to solve it. However, thanks to the efforts of several LCs who have served as change agents, the check list is now enjoying wider use. Several experiences illustrate how this has affected care for mothers and babies.

Opportunities to discuss breastfeeding management enable the LC and physician to feel that they are partners in the effort to improve breastfeeding services.

During postpartum rounds, an IBCLC identified an infant with a short frenulum, a condition that restricted range of motion of the tongue. The mother and infant were waiting to be discharged when the short frenulum was identified. With the mother's permission, the IBCLC faxed the physician a copy of the reporting form notifying him of this problem. The pediatrician phoned to ask the mother if she wanted to remain in the hospital while he arranged for a pediatric ENT to evaluate the baby or to be released and seen by the ENT as an outpatient. The mother felt supported by her care providers, and the appropriate referrals were arranged in a convenient and timely manner.

On another occasion, a pediatrician stopped the LC (BMM) in the hallway to thank her for a recent faxed report notifying him of an at-risk infant. Such opportunities to discuss breastfeeding management enable the LC and physician to feel that they are partners in the effort to improve breastfeeding services.

While use of the reporting tool has primarily been confined to the private hospitals in the Austin community, an IBCLC who works primarily with Spanish-speaking mothers at the local public hospital recently chose to incorporate the reporting form in her work with low-income clients. She plans to fax the report to each at-risk mother's WIC clinic. This may facilitate referral to Mom's Place, a breastfeeding clinic sponsored by the Texas Department of Health, where IBCLCs and peer counselors assist income-eligible clients.

Conclusion

Will the new reporting form improve continuity of care for breastfeeding mothers and babies in the Austin community? We will not know until feedback from users of the form is received following its implementation with many mother/baby pairs. However, we feel that this notification process provides a safety net to ease the transition of mothers and babies from the hospital to the community environment. Further, the notification form works in conjunction with the AAP Guidelines that recommends early follow-up for breastfeeding babies.

By targeting at-risk dyads for notification, early follow-up may be more effectively facilitated. Improved communication contributes to greater accountability within the health care system to ensure good outcomes. That was our goal in developing this tool. Implementing the tool is a necessary next step in supporting more positive outcomes for our breastfeeding clients. We encourage other clinicians to consider using the tool to determine whether it assists them in identifying need for early intervention for mothers and babies at risk for adverse breastfeeding outcomes.

References

Alper B, Manno C (1996). Dysphagia in infants and children with oral-motor deficits: assessment and management. *Seminars in Speech and Language*, 17 (4), 283-309.

American Academy of Pediatrics (1997). Breastfeeding and the use of human milk. *Pediatrics*, 100 (6), 1035-7.

Bayday N, McCann M, Williams R, Vesper E (1997). Final Report: WIC Infant Feeding Practices Study. Office of Analysis and Evaluation, Food and Consumer Service, USDA, Alexandria, VA 22302, Contract No. 53-31998-3-003.

Chapman D, Perez-Escamilla (1999). Identification of risk factors for delayed onset of lactation. *Journal of the American Dietetic Association*, 99 (4), 450-4.

Chen D, Nommsen-Rivers L, Dewey K, Lonnerdal B (1998): Stress during labor and delivery and early lactation performance. *American Journal of Clinical Nutrition*, 68 (2), 335-45.

Crowell M, Hill P, Humenick S (1994). Relationship between obstetric analgesia and time of effective breastfeeding. *Journal of Nurse-Midwifery*, 39 (3), 150-6.

Gunther M (1955). Instinct and the nursing couple. *Lancet* 1, 576-8.

Henly S, Anderson C, Avery M, Hills-Bonczyk S, Potter S, Duckett L (1995). Anemia and insufficient milk in first-time mothers. *Birth* 22 (2), 87-92.

Hill P, Aldag J, and Chatterton R (1999). Effects of pumping style on milk production in mothers of non-nursing preterm infants. *Journal of Human Lactation*, 15 (3), 209-16.

Huggins K, Petok E, Mireles O (2000). Markers of lactation insufficiency. IN *Current Issues in Clinical Lactation* K G Auerbach, 2000. Sudbury MA: Jones and Bartlett Publishers, pp. 25-35.

Hughes V, Owen J (1993). Is breast-feeding possible after breast surgery? *MCN.* The American Journal of Maternal Child Nursing 18, (4)213-7.

Hurst N (1996). Lactation after augmentation mammoplasty. *Obsetrics and Gynecology* 87 (1), 30-4.

International Board of Lactation Consultant Examiners (1999). *Code of Ethics.* Falls Church, VA: IBLCE (Principle #9).

International Lactation Consultant Association (1999). *Standards of Practice of IBCLC Lactation Consultants.* Raleigh, NC: ILCA. (Standards 1.3.6 and 2.5)

Lauwers J, Shinskie D (2000). *Counseling the Nursing Mother: A Lactation Consultant's Guide,* 3rd ed. Sudbury, MA: Jones and Bartlett Publishers, p. 484.

Livingstone V, Stringer J (1999). The treatment of *staphylococcus aureus* infected sore nipples: a randomized comparative study. *Journal of Human Lactation* 15 (3), 241-6.

McBride M, Danner S (1987). Sucking disorders in neurologically impaired infants: assessment and facilitation of breastfeeding. *Clinics in Perinatology,* 14 (1), 109-30.

Messner A, Lalakea L, Aby J, MacMahon J, Bair E (2000). Ankyloglossia: incidence and associated feeding difficulties. *Archives of Otolaryngology, Head and Neck Surgery* 126 (1), 36-9.

Neifert M (1999). Clinical aspects of lactation. *Clinics in Perinatology,* 26 (2), 281-306.

Neifert M (1996). Early assessment of the breastfeeding infant. *Contemporary Pediatrics,* 13 (10), 142-66.

Neifert M, Seacat J, Jobe W (1985). Lactation failure due to insufficient glandular development of the breast. *Pediatrics* 76 (5), 823-8.

Neubauer S, Ferris S, Chase C, Fanelli J, Thomposon C, Lammi-Keefe C, et al (1993). Delayed lactogenesis in women with insulin-dependent diabetes mellitus. *American Journal of Clinical Nutrition* 58 (1), 54-60.

Nyhan W (1952). Stool frequency of normal infants in the first week of life. *Pediatrics,* 10 (4), 414-25.

Powers N (1999). Slow weight gain and low milk supply in the breastfeeding dyad. *Clinics in Perinatology* 26 (2), 399-430.

Ramsey M, Gisel E (1996). Neonatal sucking and maternal feeding practices. *Developmental Medicine and Child Neurology,* 38 (1), 34-47.

Willis C, Livingstone V (1995). Infant insufficient milk syndrome associated with maternal postpartum hemorrhage. *Journal of Human Lactation,* 11 (2), 123-6.

Woolridge M (1986). Aetiology of sore nipples. *Midwifery,* 2, 172-6.

Fig. 1: The High Risk For Breastfeeding Problems Notification Form

Date: _____

From: Hospital Lactation Dept: _____

RE: Baby's name and DOB: _____

Mother's name/current Ph No: _____

Dear Doctor _____:

Because mothers are being discharged before their milk comes in, lactation problems may not be evident until after discharge. "Many lactation problems do not become evident until milk starts being produced in abundance and the effectiveness of milk transfer during feedings can be evaluated." M. Neifert, *Clinics in Perinatology* 1999, 26 (2), 290.

Maternal Risk Factors Noted:
- [ ] History of previous breast surgery
- [ ] Anatomic breast variations
- [ ] Minimal breast changes during pregnancy
- [ ] Medical illness _____
- [ ] Flat/inverted nipples
- [ ] Long/difficult labor—primiparous mother (associated in the medical lit. with delays in onset of copious milk production)

Infant Risk Factors Noted:
- [ ] Prematurity or Intrauterine Growth Retardation (IUGR)
- [ ] Twins or other multiples
- [ ] Jaundice
- [ ] Baby with latch-on problem
- [ ] Oral cleft and other oral anatomic variations _____
- [ ] Medical illness/neuromotor problems _____
- [ ] Loss of >7% of birthweight at discharge
- [ ] Suppl. feed by bottle/cup/SNS/other due to hypoglycemia/non-alert/separation

Community Resources for Breastfeeding:

Free phone counseling: La Leche League (accredited volunteers) Hotline # _____

Income-eligible LC services Ph: _____

Out-patient LC services at this hospital _____

Private Practice Lactation Consultants (IBCLC) _____

Developed by: Bernadette Maloney, RN, IBCLC, Valerie Mick, RN, IBCLC, and Barbara Wilson-Clay, IBCLC, 1999

May be copied freely if kept in its original form. Phone numbers and places to obtain assistance may be altered.

On Behalf of Breastfeeding

Last Step First

Diane Wiessinger, MS, IBCLC

Diane Wiessinger is a lactation consultant in private practice in Ithaca, NY, a mother of two, a La Leche League leader, and editor of this column, which focuses on breastfeeding advocacy. Contact the author at 136 Ellis Hollow Creek Road, Ithaca, NY 14850 USA.

Current Issues in Clinical Lactation, 2002, 69–73; Baby-Friendly Hospital Initiative, Ten Steps to Succesful Breastfeeding.

The "Ten Steps to Successful Breastfeeding" are the foundation of the WHO/UNICEF Baby-Friendly Hospital Initiative (BFHI). They summarize the maternity practices necessary to support breastfeeding (1998).

Step Ten: Foster the establishment of breastfeeding support groups and refer mothers to them on discharge from the hospital or clinic.

I have a few photographs of little girls, one a mere 18 months old, clutching dolls to their flat chests, shirts lifted, looking like experienced breastfeeding mothers. They are learning to breastfeed without pressure, over time, from women they want to emulate. I think these little girls represent the heart of the Baby-Friendly Hospital Initiative's Step Ten.

Michael Woolridge spoke at a breastfeeding conference (Woolridge M, [1991] "Breastfeeding in the United States and Thailand: parallels and differences." International Lactation Consultant Association Annual Conference, Session 200, Miami, Florida) of a hospital with dismal breastfeeding protocols. All babies were bottle-fed before their first breastfeeding, which occurred many hours post-birth. Rooming-in was non-existent. Breastfeedings were scheduled at widely spaced intervals. Supplementation was routine. What percentage of these mothers, he asked, were still breastfeeding several weeks after discharge? The answer was in the high nineties. They were discharged, he explained, into a breast-feeding culture. These mothers, too, represent the heart of Step Ten.

A friend of mine recently experienced first-hand the difference Step Ten can make. About six months after giving birth, she spent a Saturday at a breastfeeding support group conference. At the conference was a small sea of breastfed babies carried in slings by parents who were busily sharing experiences. The next afternoon, she went to a reunion at her birth center. The center, she emphasized, had done a wonderful job on-site–low-intervention births, consistent and accurate breastfeeding information, certified lactation consultants on staff who also offered help post-discharge. In short, they followed each of the first nine steps. But during the reunion, hers was the only child who breastfed. All but hers were in infant seats or strollers, and there was great curiosity about the novel way she carried her baby. The nurses were amazed that her child was still exclusively breastfeeding. What had happened to those wonderful beginnings? Was it simply that these mothers had been discharged into a large, anonymous, bottle-feeding city to rely on the role models they found there? My friend found different role models—without the help of the birth center. She found a breastfeeding "mini-culture" to sustain her in a larger bottle-feeding society.

A mini-culture of breastfeeding role models is important both before and after a woman begins breastfeeding. "Lact-net" is an international e-mail user group for breastfeeding specialists, most of whom consider themselves "allied health professionals." Yet when the group topic turned to why the participants themselves decided to breastfeed, only half had based their decision on health issues. The other half mentioned role models—family members, friends, even a stranger on a bus. That finding alone should be surprising when we think of how vigorously we promote breastfeeding as a health issue but with how little emphasis we give the relationship.

The differences among the Lactnet comments were equally revealing. "I decided I would try to breastfeed for six months" was typical of a health-reason respondent, the language of a woman thinking about limits and possible failure. Those whose decisions were role model-based were more likely to say something open-ended and enthusiastic: "I knew that was how I wanted to raise my children."

The Ten Steps are written in chronological order from a hospital perspective. They pro-

The Ten Steps are written in chronological order from a hospital perspective. They proceed with institutional logic from written policy through staff training to delivery to the early days of breastfeeding—each step equally important in its own time, each growing out of the step before.

ceed with institutional logic from written policy through staff training to delivery to the early days of breastfeeding—each step equally important in its own time, each growing out of the step before. Following this logic, Step Ten is in its proper post-discharge position. Yet because of the sequence, it is easy to assume that the last step is also the least important. And, many hospital staff—including lactation consultants!—neglect it altogether.

But imagine what might result if a hospital *began* its efforts by establishing a breastfeeding support group or by enthusiastically promoted an existing one in the community. Imagine that it strongly encouraged everyone who planned a birth at that facility to attend at least one or

A mini-culture of breastfeeding role models is important both before and after a woman begins breastfeeding.

two support group meetings beforehand, and made sure each mother knew at discharge when the next meeting occurred—before it addressed the other nine steps.

Imagine the pregnant woman's experience at that group. She would return home knowing not only a support group phone number but also at least one face and personality to match. She might leave pondering her first-ever sight of a nursing toddler, or the vision of a baby falling asleep at breast. She might have seen a mother playing nursing games with her baby—toes-in-the-mouth, or peekaboo-with-the-shirt, mother and baby smiling at one another—and said to herself, "That's how I want to look in a few months." She might not have learned about alveoli or oxytocin, but she might have a clearer image of her baby staying at her side following the birth. After discharge, sore, uncertain again after (let's suppose) a truly frightful hospital experience, she could return to a group of familiar faces who would gather around and say, "We remember you! It's tough right now, isn't it? It gets better." How very different from having one neatly dressed (or white-coated) LC answer her questions in an office or over the phone!

I remember a well-educated client, a speech pathologist with a specialty in geriatric problems. No amount of reassurance on my part gave her confidence that her baby's squeaks and gurgles were normal. They were, after all, the very sounds about which she warned her nursing-home students. I invited her to a breastfeeding support group. The dozen or so mothers all nodded calmly when she described the sounds: "Yes, our babies do that, too. Maybe it's because they can't clear their throats." They showed the same calm unanimity over several other anxious questions she asked: "Yes, our babies spit up sometimes. It looks like a lot, doesn't it? Especially on a mother-in-law!" "Yes, our babies often want to nurse within minutes of seeming full. We don't know why. More nursing seems to work." Afterwards, my client told me, "You know, I was going from here straight to the doctor's. Now I think I'll just go home and enjoy my baby."

Once a month is too long to wait for this kind of group reassurance, but not all facilities can manage a weekly group. Perhaps the most important service monthly support groups provide is a place for women to form like-minded "play groups"—friendships that can sustain women from week to week.

A mother in one such group arrived with chronic milk supply problems, a grim expression, and a goal of "toughing it out" for four months if she could. She sat on a couch next to another woman with the same problem who was relaxing into motherhood with her older baby. After only two weekly meetings, the newer mother felt like Superwoman (laughingly making muscles at me to prove it). She nursed happily into her baby's toddlerhood, having finally grasped that breastfeeding is Much More Than Milk. I had given her technical support and encouragement, but it was a tousled, sleep-deprived role model who helped her feel competent.

Maybe you don't care for your local support group options. Get over it.

Maybe you don't care for your local support group options. Get over it. . . .It will be a glorious day when we can afford infighting. We're not there yet.

Go to the meetings. Get to know the group's leaders. Find your common ground. And if common ground doesn't exist, create it. Step Ten is simply too important to fail from personality conflicts or mutual misunderstanding or a fear of competition or turf invasion. Embrace Step Ten *and the people who make it work in your area.* Learn from each other. You and your facility are a full ten percent short of being Baby-Friendly if you don't, and all your institutional successes may not compensate for this one failure. It will be a glorious day when we can afford infighting. We're not there yet.

Mothers want to "do it right." They train for it from toddlerhood, whether by clutching dolls to their chests or by inserting pointy plastic bottles into round plastic mouths. And for all but the most determined, "doing it right" probably means adhering to a role model. By making sure that Step Ten is given at least as much weight as the other nine steps, *any* facility can establish an ongoing mini-culture where mothers can find the breastfeeding role models they need.

The last of the Ten Steps doesn't involve a checklist or a protocol. It resists careful planning. It is determinedly non-medical. But it is breastfeeding support in its oldest, most endur-ing form—women learning without pressure, over time, from women they want to emulate. Step Ten is the medical model deferring to the role model. And I think it should come first.

Reference

World Health Organization, (1998). *Evidence for the Ten Steps to Successful Breastfeeding*. Geneva: Division of Child Health and Development (WHO/CHD/98.9), p.5.

Index to CICL - 2002

Instructions to Authors

Current Issues in Clinical Lactation

Current Issues in Clinical Lactation (CICL) publishes evaluation of reports deriving from clinical human lactation and research discussions of the clinical experiences of lactation specialists/consultants/scientists. Case reports and case series, and the business aspects of assisting breastfeeding mothers and babies, also are published.

COVER LETTER—Submit each manuscript with a cover letter containing the following language:

"The contents of this manuscript are my/our original work and have not been published, in whole or in part, prior to or simultaneous with my/our submission of the manuscript to *CICL*. I/We acknowledge that simultaneous submission of the manuscript to more than one journal will result in automatic rejection for publication in *CICL*.

In consideration of the action of Editor(s) and Jones and Bartlett Publishers, Inc. in reviewing and editing my/our submission entitled _____, the undersigned contributor(s) hereby transfer, assign, and otherwise convey exclusively to *CICL*, its successors and assigns, all copyright ownership in the event that such work is published in *CICL*. I/We acknowledge that Editor(s) of *CICL* and Jones and Bartlett Publishers are under no obligation to publish this manuscript. It is my/our understanding that said copyright ownership will revert to me/us if the manuscript is not published in *CICL*.

I/WE EXPRESSLY COVENANT, WARRANT AND REPRESENT THAT:

This manuscript does not infringe on any copyright. If copyrighted material is included in the manuscript, I/we have secured written permission for its publication in *CICL*.

This manuscript is delivered to *CICL* free from any claims of any nature whatsoever and its publication will not subject Editor(s) or Jones and Bartlett Publishers to claims for payment to any third party.

I/We have the full right, power and authority to make this agreement and to grant the rights herein granted."

Manuscripts without cover letters including such language will be returned without review. *Each author/ contributor must sign and date* the cover letter containing the above language.

ALL SUBMISSIONS exclusive of letters—Send the original and four copies including all tables and illustrations, typed double-spaced on white bond 8 1/2″ × 11″ with 1″ margins. Number all pages consecutively. Authors should retain one copy. A fax or e-mail acknowledgment of receipt will be sent. For a posted acknowledgment of receipt, enclose a self-addressed, (and stamped, if from USA) envelope.

Standard written English usage and syntax are expected. APA style preferences will be observed. Titles should be concise and clear. Do not use slang, medical jargon, or obscure abbreviations or phrasing. Metric measurement is preferred; equivalent English measurement may be included in parentheses. Use generic names for drugs or devices; put trade names in parentheses.

See Manuscript Submission Checklist for specifics of format.

Type *references* on separate page, listed alphabetically. Limit references to 20 primary sources, preferably no older than 5 years. Reviews/historical manuscripts may contain more than 20 references. Cite all quotations, previous study findings, and facts the reader may question. Use the following style:

- Journal (list first six authors, followed by et al):
Hill PD, Humenick SS, Brennan ML, Woolley D (1997). Does early supplementation affect long-term breastfeeding? *Clinical Pediatrics 36* (6), 345-50.

- Book (single author or set of authors for entire volume):
Van Esterik P (1989). *Beyond the Breast-Bottle Controversy* (pp. 20-27). New Brunswick, NJ: Rutgers University Press.

- Book (edited volume with several authors of chapters):
Riordan J (1999). Child health (Chapter 19): In J Riordan, KG Auerbach, *Breastfeeding and Human Lactation* (2nd ed.) (pp. 601-36). Boston: Jones and Bartlett Publishers.

- Unpublished works (conference presentations, Masters or Doctoral theses, and manuscripts that are *in press*). Provide author(s) name(s), title, source, date of presentation/degree conferral.

- Personal Communications and all other unpublished materials: Include *only* in the body of the manuscript.

Tables must be clear to the reader without referring to the text. Type each table, with a descriptive title, on a separate page, following the text and references pages. Identify where in the manuscript each table should be placed.

Key words and Pull Quotes: List up to 5 key words for use in indexing. Provide up to 3 pull quotes that identify a) the primary outcome of the research study or discussion, b) the major reason for addressing the topic, c) the primary implication for clinicians in lactation practice.

Illustrations should be unmounted black ink drawings or black and white glossy photographs. Label each illustration on its back, and include the author's name and "top". Identify where in the manuscript each illustration should be placed. Do not staple, clip together, mount, or trim prints.

Photographs of subjects must be accompanied by signed written consent from the subject and/or the minor's parent or guardian. If using a published figure, provide written permission for use from the copyright holder; acknowledge source in a footnote.

Photos for "Clinical Observation Highlight" should be sent to the Editorial office with the clinical question and sufficient information to explain the problem pictured and how the concern was resolved.

Review Process - All submissions with the exception of Letters are anonymously reviewed by at least three reviewers. Rejected manuscripts will be returned to the author(s).

Clinical Practice Discussions - Limit manuscripts to 8 pages, exclusive of table pages and references pages. List up to five (5) keywords for indexing. The manuscript should include an *abstract* no longer than 100 words, including clinical issue/problem, and key recommendation for other practitioners; *introduction* including a brief discussion of relevant literature; *discussion* of implications of the clinical issue/problem; *implications* and *recommendations* for the lactation practitioner.

Research Studies and Commentaries - Limit manuscripts to 12 pages, exclusive of table pages and references pages. List up to five (5) key words for indexing. The manuscript should include an *abstract* no longer than 100 words, including purpose, method, and results; *introduction*; description of the *methods*, including the technique and observations or data obtained, where appropriate; *results* obtained where appropriate; and a brief *discussion* of the importance of the findings. To distinguish between infant feeding groups, see Labbok M, Krasovec K, (1990). Toward consistency in breastfeeding definitions. *Studies in Family Planning 21* (2), 226-30.

"The Business of Clinical Practice" must contain sufficient information for the reader to identify the business problem presented. Authors should include a brief *introduction* of the problem, *how* it was *identified*, its *resolution* (if any), and *recommendations* for other clinicians.

Research Notes, "Breastfeeding Notes", and Case Presentations must contain sufficient information for the reader to understand those elements supporting the outcome. Authors should include a brief *introduction*, including review of the relevant literature, *history* of the problem, the *research question/case presentation* including outcome (if appropriate), and *recommenda-*

tions regarding future investigations and/or assistance in future situations. Client confidentiality must be protected in the presentation.

Contact the Editorial Office with questions pertaining to proposed submissions.

LETTERS TO THE EDITOR - Only signed letters no longer than 400 words will be published. Letters longer than 400 words may be edited or considered for "Breastfeeding Notes."

MANUSCRIPT SUBMISSION CHECK LIST
Please submit a copy of this checklist with the appropriate elements noted to verify that your submission is complete.

General
___ Original and 4 copies
___ Typed double-spaced on one side only, 1″ margin on 8 1/2″ × 11″
___ Order of pages: Title page, abstract, body of paper, references, tables, figures, photographs
___ Cover letter with copyright assignment statement, date and signature of each author
___ Consent to photograph (if applicable)
___ A self-addressed (if in USA, stamped) envelope for acknowledgment of receipt
___ Computer disk (Format of 6.0 or lower *only*). Software format is _____
___ Copy of this checklist, appropriately marked

Title Page
___ Full title of manuscript
___ Author(s) name(s) and degrees; up to three sets of initials per author
___ Name and complete address for communications pertaining to this submission
___ Daytime and evening phone numbers
___ FAX and E-mail address of senior author
___ Funding source (if applicable)
___ Brief (1-2 sentence) biographical note about each author

___ Up to 5 keywords
___ Up to 3 pull quotes

Abstract
___ Title of manuscript
___ No more than 100 words
___ Include purpose, findings/recommendations, conclusion(s)

Body of Manuscript
___ Introduction
___ Aim and Methods (if applicable)
___ Sample Population (if applicable)
___ Definition of feeding groups (if applicable)
___ Findings/Observations
___ Conclusions
___ Limitations (if applicable)
___ Implications for clinical practice and/or future research (if applicable)

References
___ Identified in text by author and year
___ Typed double-spaced, alphabetically, on separate sheet(s)
___ Style and punctuation of references follow format illustrated in these instructions

Table, Figures
___ Typed double-spaced on separate sheets
___ Placement in manuscript is identified
___ Copy of permission to reprint (if applicable); acknowledgment of original published sources footnoted

Photographs
___ For each photo submission, copy of permission to photograph (all subjects; adult signs for any minors pictured)
___ Placement in manuscript is identified

Send ALL submissions to:
CICL Editorial Office
ATTENTION: KG Auerbach, PhD, IBCLC
6145 N. Beulah Avenue
Ferndale, WA 98248-9381 USA

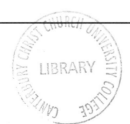

Core Curriculum for Lactation Consultant Practice
Marsha Walker, RN, IBCLC
© 2002, ISBN: 0-7637-1038-5, Paper, Price: $44.95

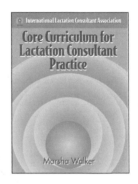

Based on the IBLCE exam blueprint, this new resource allows aspiring and established lactation consultants to assess their knowledge, experience, and expertise in developing an effective study plan for certification. Those who contributed to this text bring a wealth of knowledge and experience into a forum designed to ultimately benefit the mothers, babies, and families to whom lactation consultants are responsible.

Comprehensive Lactation Consultant Exam Review
Linda J. Smith, BSE, FACCE, IBCLC
© 2001, ISBN: 0-7637-0920-4, Paper, Price: $53.95

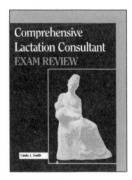

Comprehensive Lactation Consultant Exam Review parallels the 13 content areas of the IBLCE examination, making it the perfect study guide for examination and recertification candidates, breastfeeding/lactation specialists, dietitians, childbirth educators, nurses, and breastfeeding counselors. The companion CD-ROM contains 240 full color clinical pictures.

Prices subject to change.

Counseling the Nursing Mother: A Lactation Consultant's Guide, Third Edition
Judith Lauwers, BA, IBCLC
Debbie Shinskie, RN, IBCLC
© 2000, ISBN: 0-7637-0975-1, Hardcover, Price: $57.95

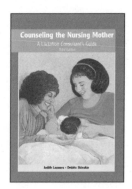

With enlightening historical and cultural perspectives on breastfeeding, *Counseling the Nursing Mother* takes great care to introduce and explain the complete spectrum of the lactation consultant profession. Major issues addressed include prenatal concerns through weaning, maternal health, and nutrition.

Pocket Guide for Counseling the Nursing Mother
Debbie Shinskie, RN, IBCLC
Judith Lauwers, BA, IBCLC
© 2002, ISBN: 0-7637-1820-3, Paper, Price: $24.95

Convenient and functional, *Pocket Guide for Counseling the Nursing Mother* will help lactation consultants establish partnerships with mothers to build confidence and self-esteem and provide an effective learning environment to actively involve mothers in problem-solving and decision-making.

Clinical Lactation: A Visual Guide
Kathleen G. Auerbach, PhD, IBCLC
Jan Riordan, EdD, RN, IBCLC, FAAN
© 2000, ISBN: 0-7637-0919-0, Paper, Price: $41.95

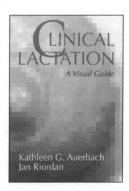

This invaluable resource prepares clinicians for practice by enabling them to evaluate photographs of both overt and subtle differences in clinical presentations.

Prices subject to change.

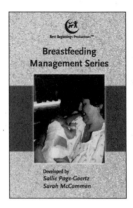
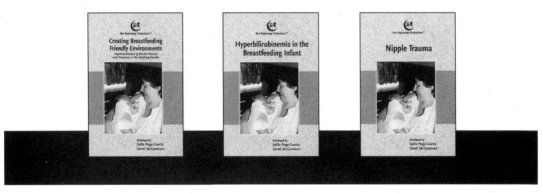

Breastfeeding and Human Lactation, Second Edition

Jan Riordan, EdD, RN, IBCLC, FAAN
Kathleen G. Auerbach, PhD, IBCLC
© 1999, ISBN: 0-7637-0545-4, Hardcover, Price: $93.95

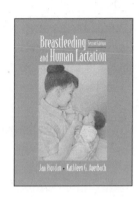

The second edition of *Breastfeeding and Human Lactation* is the most comprehensive reference available to nurses, nurse midwives, lactation consultants, childbirth educators, dietitians, and all other professionals who provide direct service to breastfeeding families. It offers information on clinical management of breastfeeding, maternal nutrition, care plans, breastfeeding promotion, and more.

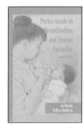

Pocket Guide to Breastfeeding and Human Lactation, Second Edition

Jan Riordan, EdD, RN, IBCLC, FAAN
Kathleen G. Auerbach, PhD, IBCLC
© 2001, ISBN: 0-7637-1469-0, Paper, Price: $24.95

This quick and easy reference answers clinical questions about breastfeeding and covers topics such as medications, birth control, maternal infections, breast lumps, and mastitis.

Also available:

Study Guide for Breastfeeding and Human Lactation, Second Edition
Jan Riordan, EdD, RN, IBCLC, FAAN
Kathleen G. Auerbach, PhD, IBCLC
© 1999, ISBN: 0-7637-0829-1, Paper, Price: $24.95

Resource Guide to Accompany Breastfeeding and Human Lactation
Jan Riordan, EdD, RN, IBCLC, FAAN
Kathleen G. Auerbach, PhD, IBCLC
© 1997, ISBN: 0-7637-0220-X, Paper, Price: $42.95

Prices subject to change.

Coach's Notebook: Games and Strategies for Lactation Education
Linda J. Smith, BSE, FACCE, IBCLC
© 2002, ISBN: 0-7637-1819-X, Paper, Price: $35.95

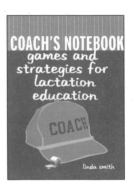

Contains a wide variety of games and activities for teaching breastfeeding and human lactation, each of which has been tried, tested, and refined by the author and other educators. For each game you'll find goals, ideal audiences, times to play, and specific instructions for making teaching and learning human lactation fun and informative.

Lactation Specialist Self Study Series
Rebecca Black, MS, RD/LD, IBCLC
Leasa Jarman, MS
Jan Simpson, RN, BSN, IBCLC
© 1998, ISBN: 0-7637-1974-9, Paper,
Price: $157.95

This self-directed learning series is designed to assist the learner in studying the field of lactation in a systematic fashion. Modules include ample illustrations, reference lists, and multiple choice review questions for assessment of learning. Continuing education credits are available from credentialing organizations in the lactation, nursing, and dietetic professions.

- **Module 1: The Support of Breastfeeding**
  © 1998, ISBN: 0-7637-0208-0, Paper, Price: $43.95

- **Module 2: The Process of Breastfeeding**
  © 1998, ISBN: 0-7637-0195-5, Paper, Price: $43.95

- **Module 3: The Science of Breastfeeding**
  © 1998, ISBN: 0-7637-0194-7, Paper, Price: $43.95

- **Module 4: The Management of Breastfeeding**
  © 1998, ISBN: 0-7637-0193-9, Paper, Price: $43.95

Prices subject to change.

Lamaze™ International Supports Breastfeeding

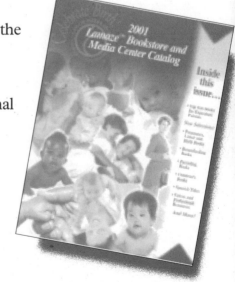

Breastfeeding is natural and simple, but support and understanding are essential for women to be successful breastfeeders in today's world. The Lamaze Breastfeeding Support Specialist Workshop is designed for those individuals who wish to improve their ability to enhance the initiation and duration of breastfeeding:

- Childbirth Educators
- Hospital or community based health professionals
- Individuals interested in pursuing certification as Lactation Consultants
- Women who want to support other women both prenatally and during the early post partum period.

This workshop is offered at locations nationwide, or contact Lamaze International to bring it to your community.

Select books and other items on breastfeeding, childbirth and early parenting for professionals and parents. Visit the Lamaze Bookstore and Media Center online at **www.lamaze.org**.

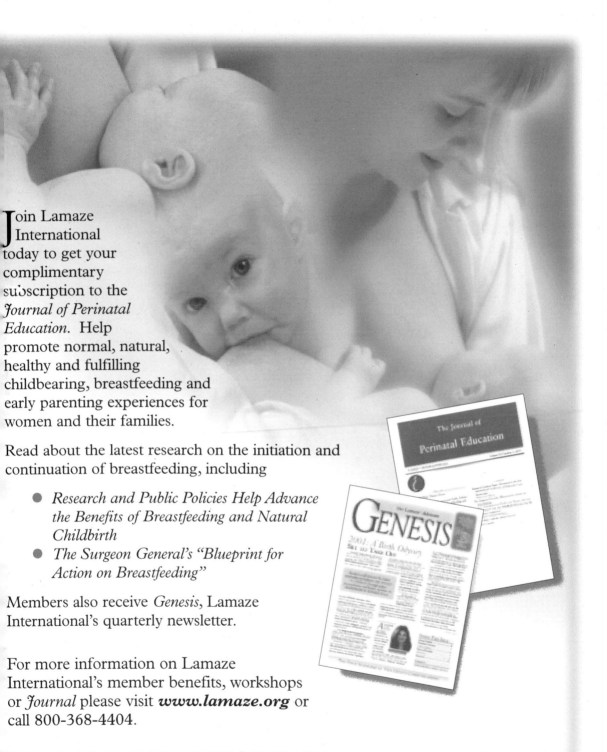